THE BRITISH
MEDICAL ASSOCIATION

CARER'S
MANUAL

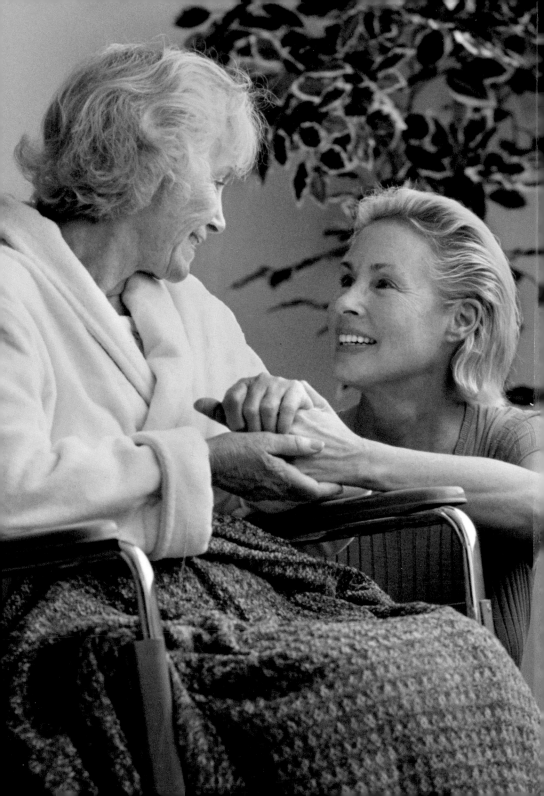

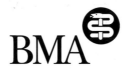

BMA

THE BRITISH
MEDICAL ASSOCIATION

CARER'S
MANUAL

**LONDON, NEW YORK, MELBOURNE,
MUNICH, AND DELHI**

BRITISH MEDICAL ASSOCIATION
Chair of Council Dr. Mark Porter
Treasurer Dr. Andrew Dearden
Chairman of Representative Body Dr. Steve Hajioff
BMA Consulting Medical Editor Dr. Michael Peters MB BS

CONTRIBUTORS
Russell Caller, Helen Crawley, Jemima Dunne,
Anna Jordan, Polly Landsberg, Dawn Mohun,
Henny Pearmain, David Taylor

DK
Senior editors Janet Mohun, Andrea Bagg
Project art editor Duncan Turner
Editors Joanna Edwards, Martyn Page
Editorial assistance Kaiya Shang
DK picture library Sue Peachy, Rob Nunn
Producer, pre-production Nikoleta Parasaki
Senior producer Alice Sykes
Jacket editor Manisha Majithia
Jacket designer Mark Cavanagh
Jacket manager Sophia Tampakopoulos
Managing editor Angeles Gavira
Managing art editor Michelle Baxter
Art Director Philip Ormerod
Publisher Sarah Larter
Associate publishing director Liz Wheeler
Publishing director Jonathan Metcalf

Art direction Nigel Wright, XAB
Photography Ruth Jenkinson

DK INDIA
Editor Ritu Mishra
Art Editor Shreya Anand Virmani
DTP designers Arjinder Singh, Bimlesh Tiwary
Managing editor Rohan Sinha
Deputy managing art editor Sudakshina Basu
Production manager Pankaj Sharma
DTP manager Balwant Singh

First published in Great Britain in 2013
by Dorling Kindersley Limited
80 Strand, London WC2R 0RL
Penguin Group (UK)

2 4 6 8 10 9 7 5 3 1
001 – 183051 – June 2013

IMPORTANT READER NOTICE

The BMA Carer's Manual provides information on many aspects
of caring for someone at home. The book is not a substitute
for expert medical advice, however, and you are advised
always to consult a doctor or other health professional
for specific information on personal health matters. Never disregard
expert medical advice or delay in seeking advice or treatment due
to information obtained from this book. The naming of any product,
treatment, or organization in this book does not imply endorsement
by the BMA, BMA Consulting Medical Editor, other consultants or
contributors, or publisher, nor does the omission
of any such names indicate disapproval. The BMA, BMA Consulting
Medical Editor, consultants, contributors, and publisher do not accept
any legal responsibility for any personal injury
or other damage or loss arising from any use or misuse
of the information and advice in this book.

This book uses he and she in alternate chapters to describe the person
being cared for, except when a specific person is being shown in a
photograph. This is for clarity and convenience and does not reflect a
preference for either sex.

A CIP catalogue record for this book is available from the
British Library.

ISBN 9 781 4093 2082 1
Printed and bound in China by Leo Paper Products LTD

See our complete catalogue at
www.dk.com

CONTENTS

FOREWORD

In the past few years there has been a huge increase in the number of people who care for loved ones – be they partners, relatives, or friends – at home. There are many reasons for this – hospitals tend to discharge patients sooner, people are generally living longer, and many people simply cannot afford private professional care. For a new carer, the prospect of looking after someone who may be elderly or have health problems can seem daunting, not only because of the responsibility involved and the practical issues, but also because of the disruption to normal life.

There are many sources of information about various different aspects of caring – so many, in fact, that it can be difficult to know where to start and which sources give reliable information. This book aims to provide a single, authoritative guide to all the important aspects of home caring. There are chapters with practical advice about adapting the home, diet and eating, social and mental wellbeing, aiding mobility, comfort in bed, personal care, nursing techniques, first aid emergencies, and end-of-life care. There is also

information about legal and financial matters, and useful resources.

One important but often overlooked aspect of caring is the physical and mental wellbeing of the carer him- or herself. Caring can be physically and emotionally demanding, and it can be difficult to adjust to changed relationships, not only with the person being cared for but also with other family members, friends, and colleagues. There is also the risk that the carer may become so involved in the practical everyday tasks of caring that his or her own health suffers. This book provides guidance on how to cope with these issues – and how to get help and support, if necessary – so that the process of caring is as stress-free as possible.

Everybody and every situation is different so inevitably this book cannot substitute for advice specifically tailored for you and the person you are caring for. However, I believe that the information here will provide a sound foundation for caring for a loved one – and yourself – and will help to make caring a rewarding experience for both of you.

Dr. Michael Peters
BMA Consulting Medical Editor

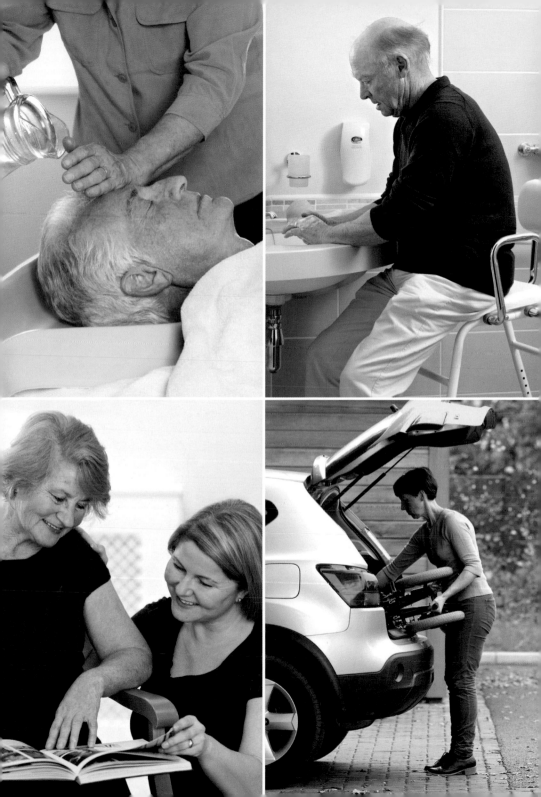

1

BECOMING A CARER

■ ROLE OF THE CARER ■ DECIDING TO BECOME A CARER
■ LIVING ARRANGEMENTS ■ CHANGED RELATIONSHIPS
■ LOOKING AFTER YOURSELF ■ YOUR EMOTIONAL WELLBEING
■ GETTING HELP AND SUPPORT

THE ROLE OF THE CARER

Being a carer means taking responsibility for another person – caring for her health and welfare with compassion, respect, and dignity. If a close relative, spouse, partner, or friend is elderly or becomes ill, you may be the person best placed to offer her the highest quality care. You are likely to know her well and she will probably trust you more than anyone.

Being in a caring role requires patience and a fine balance between promoting independence and providing help when needed. Sometimes taking on this role may not be the best option, either for you or for the person who needs care, and it is important to look realistically at the person's full needs as well as at your own. You should also consider the needs of other members of your family.

Levels of care

The amount of care you need to give will depend on the capabilities of the person you are looking after. Some people may just require extra help with daily activities, such as cooking or shopping. Or someone you are caring for outside the home may need occasional help to attend hospital appointments or a community support group for elderly people.

WHY CARE MIGHT BE NEEDED

- **General decline in health and fitness** Most elderly people live independent lives for the greater part of their lives and enjoy their latter years in relatively good and stable health. However, some decline in health and fitness is an inevitable part of the normal aging process, and help with daily care may eventually be needed.

- **Memory loss** Some short-term memory loss, such as forgetting where the keys are, affects everyone as they get older. However, the severe memory loss that occurs with dementia (see panel, opposite) may make it unsafe for the person to live alone any more. This may be because she forgets to turn the gas hob off, or she forgets where she has parked her car, or she may go out for a walk to the local shops and suddenly forget how to get back home.

- **Illness** Many illnesses, such as stroke, heart attack, cancer, and dementia, may mean that a person needs care. Many such illnesses are more common in elderly people and, when combined with the natural age-related decline in abilities, means their health needs can be complex. However, younger people can suffer from such illnesses, too.

- **Falls** Elderly people are more likely to fall than those who are younger, and if they do so they are more likely to injure themselves. Falls also have a damaging psychological impact on older people, leading to loss of confidence, fear, and restriction of activities. Combined with the problems that an elderly person might already have, a fall may be the "tipping point" between independent living and the need for care.

- **Depression and anxiety** These conditions are more common in elderly people as they become less able and lose their life role or independence. Depression can also be a result of medical conditions, such as low thyroid activity or a heart problem, which are more common in elderly people.

- **Bereavement** If an elderly person loses a life partner, this leads to a great sense of loss and grief and, for some, the feeling that life now has no meaning. It can also throw out the balance of the person's life as the life skills and health needs of two elderly people often complement each other – when one person dies, the person left may find it hard to cope.

- **Chronic disabling illness** People with long-term progressive illnesses, such as multiple sclerosis (MS) and Parkinson's disease, will need varying levels of care, depending on the severity and stage of the illness.

However, if a person requires help with more basic needs, such as feeding or bathing, you may need to give 24-hour care. In these circumstances, if the person does not already live with, you may need to consider having her move in with you. Adaptations to the home may be required (pp.28–41). Alternatively, a care home may need to be considered.

■ **Short-term care** Your relative, spouse, partner, or friend might just need short-term care while she recovers from an accident, such as a fall, or from surgery or sudden illness, such as a heart attack. While initially she may need intensive care in hospital, once she starts to recover, care at home is probably the best option.

She may need full care initially and, if she is not already living with you, you may want to consider moving into her home on a short-term basis. As she improves and gains strength, your caring role will gradually diminish. Eventually, you should be able to return to your own home but continue to visit as needed.

■ **Long-term care** A person who has permanent loss of physical or mental abilities will need long-term care. Such deterioration can come on gradually and may not be obvious at first. You may notice that the person loses confidence in going

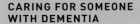
CARING FOR SOMEONE WITH DEMENTIA

The onset of dementia is a very common reason for a person needing regular care. Many people are now living well into their 80s and 90s, and dementia can set in while they are still in good physical health. If you are caring for someone diagnosed with dementia, it is important to realize that it can be a degenerative and long-term disease. The problems resulting from dementia are wide and variable and include the following:

■ Memory difficulties are one of the major symptoms in dementia, and lead to a range of problems, such as forgetting to turn off a flame or getting lost when out.

■ Reduced physical coordination can make it more difficult to control movement.

■ Impaired balance makes it harder for a person to react if she stumbles or bends over to pick up a dropped object, making falls more likely.

■ Disturbed sleep is common and may be due to bad dreams, night wanderings, or night-time hallucinations (p.107). Daytime drowsiness as a result of poor sleep may mean that the person forgets to eat or drink.

out or driving, and perhaps has less interest in hobbies than previously. If the person is living in her own home, you may notice that the general running of the house, such as cleaning and paying bills, is falling behind. If she is living with you, her need for increased care may become obvious if, for example, you are reluctant to leave her alone while you go out to the shops or if you feel that going to work for a full day is too long to safely leave her.

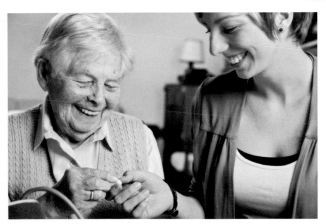

A helping hand
A gradual loss of dexterity can be extremely debilitating as it can affect everything from doing up a button to handling medication. Help in these tasks may often be required.

DECIDING TO BECOME A CARER

If your partner or spouse needs caring for, your role as her carer may have developed gradually and not been one that you consciously chose. If a friend or relative not living with you needs care, the decision to take on this role is not one you should make alone. Talk it over with family members as well as the person who is now in need of care. Also consult the person's doctor, who can arrange for assessment of her needs.

Working arrangements

It can be difficult to care for someone when you are also working. However, most workers have statutory rights, including the right to request flexible working hours, although employers are not obliged to agree, and the right to unpaid leave in emergencies (p.211). Your employer may also be able to offer you a sabbatical so

that you can take a career break with the certainty that your job will be kept open. You could also consider talking to your employer about the possibility of part-time work. However, these decisions are at your employer's discretion.

Your family life

Before you make the decision to care for someone outside the home, you need to consider how others in your household may be affected. Will you still have enough time to devote to the rest of the family? It's important that you discuss the situation, examining the pros and cons, and come to a decision together.

Talking to the person needing care

What does the person want? It may be that she can recognize which activities of daily living she needs support with. Having her consent to, and approval of, your help will make your role easier. If not, you may need to be more creative in how you introduce more care, for example by increasing the cleaner's hours or building more visits into your week or day.

If the person is starting to have memory problems, you may need to consider applying for power of attorney (p.213) so that you can make decisions for her if the need arises – eventually, she may lose the capacity to make her own decisions.

Community care assessment

In the UK, anyone being cared for is entitled to have a needs assessment, also called a community care assessment, to assess her strengths, abilities, and needs. To arrange an assessment contact the social services department or ask the person's doctor to refer you. The assessment may recommend help from a care assistant

---

PRACTICAL CONSIDERATIONS

You will need to consider some practical questions before you decide that you can care for your relative or friend.

- How much help is she realistically going to need?
- Am I the best person to give her the care, or could someone else help?
- Who does she want to be looked after by (if there is an option)?
- Have I discussed the situation with my immediate family and others?
- Am I going to need to adapt my home or the home of the person I am caring for?
- How will I be a part-time or full-time carer if I am still working?
- Am I prepared to give up work, if necessary?
- Am I fully aware of which benefits I may be entitled to as a carer and how these will affect my financial situation (pp.210–211)?

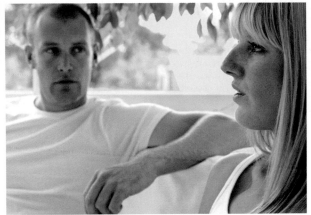

includes questions such as: What is the risk associated with the person living at home? Could she fall again? Has there been weight loss and associated weakness due to reduced appetite? If necessary, the person will be referred to a falls clinic or a memory clinic. If dementia seems to be affecting the person's safety or quality of life, she may be referred to a psycho-geriatrician.

Support network
Becoming a carer will impact on many people, and it is important to make sure that all involved are fully supportive of you and the situation.

(p.22) or that aids and adaptations are fitted to the person's home (pp.28–41). Usually a social worker will visit the person's home to do the assessment. He or she will talk to both you and the person being cared for and will carry out a series of so-called risk assessments. This

Reassessing the situation

The condition of the person you are caring for may improve, but it may not or it may become worse. If after a few weeks or months you realize that the person is not improving, you may need to reassess your original decision to care for her. Talk to her doctor, and possibly ask for a referral to a geriatrician. A care home may be the best option. For information on care home options and funding, see pp. 214 and 211.

HEALTH PROFESSIONALS

- **Doctor** The doctor of the person you are caring for can provide general medical advice and also give a referral to other medical services.

- **District nurses** These nurses can offer day-to-day day nursing help, such as changing dressings and administering injections for diabetes. They decide whether to request any other specialist nurse or care assistant to help you, and they also liaise closely with the doctor of the person's doctor.

- **Specialist nurses** There are various nurses trained to deal with particular illnesses. For example, Admiral nurses are specialist mental health nurses who provide practical and emotional support to carers of people with dementia, while Macmillan nurses provide care and support to cancer sufferers and their families.

- **Occupational therapists** They can advise on any adaptations needed for the home or specialist equipment that can help a person to stay more independent.

- **Physiotherapists** They help people to develop or maintain their physical skills by assisting them to improve their posture and movement.

- **Geriatricians** These specialist doctors help in assessing and treating elderly people with long-term disorders. Psycho-geriatricians specialize in treating those with disorders such as dementia in which mental health issues are a major factor.

- **Other health professionals** These include chiropodists or podiatrists for foot care, opticians for eye care, dentists for teeth, and dieticians for advice on eating. The person's doctor can refer her.

LIVING ARRANGEMENTS

Caring for someone who is living with you, such as your spouse, means that you are there to offer help if needed. Caring for someone outside the home brings different challenges. It is easiest to care for the person if you live close by, but with careful planning it is still possible to offer care from a distance. If someone needs help with many daily activities or it is not safe for her to live alone, you may need to consider having her move in with you.

Caring for someone in her home

Most people who need care prefer to stay in their own home among familiar possessions and surroundings. This may be possible If someone requires only part-time care, for example help with specific tasks such as shopping. She should have a community care assessment (p.12) to make sure that it is not dangerous for her to live alone.

Elderly people living alone often allow their surroundings to become cluttered with furniture or piles of papers, and this can increase the risk of falls. An occupational therapist (OT) can suggest how to help make the environment safe. The OT can also suggest what adaptations could be made to the person's home (pp.28–41) to enable her to continue living there for as long as possible. If leaving someone after your visit worries you, you could consider installing a telecare system (opposite).

Caring from a distance

Living a long distance from the person you care for can make it much harder to have the right kind of input when it is needed and makes caring a more challenging responsibility. Getting to the person in a hurry if she becomes unwell may be

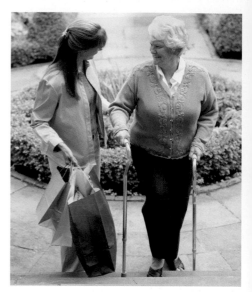

Home delivery
Many people who need some care can continue to stay in their own homes as long as they get some help with daily tasks, such as shopping.

difficult and you may be under additional financial strain as travel can be expensive, especially when you have to do it regularly. Looking after the person effectively as she ages will be challenging.

It helps to consider an organized and planned pattern of care with as many people as you need to help provide support. There may be a point when it is sensible to consider either moving closer or asking the person if she would consider moving in with you, or at least closer to where you live. Using a telecare system can take a lot of worry away from living at a distance. Try to arrange for a community assessment in the area where the person lives because she may be entitled to a care assistant (p.22) during your absence. You may prefer to find someone yourself. An Attendance Allowance (p.206) can help pay for this.

Moving in with you

Making the decision for a person to move in with you is not one to be taken lightly. First of all, ask yourself how well you and your family get on with the person now. If the answer is not very well, then having that person in your house 24 hours a day will soon become very difficult.

Other things to consider are: how much privacy you, your family, and the person you are caring for will have; whether she will be able to carry on with her own interests and entertain her own friends; and whether she will eat all her meals with the family or cook for herself sometimes. If you have young or teenage children, will she be able to cope with the noise and mess? Discuss all these issues with everybody before making a commitment.

You'll also need to consider whether adaptations to your home may be necessary, what costs are involved, and whether you can get financial help. Caring for someone in your home is demanding, and it is important that you get the help you need (pp.22–25).

Telecare and home call systems

A telecare system consists of various wireless sensors in the home that can detect if there is a problem and send an alert to a call centre. Home call systems are similar, but are intended for use by a live-in carer so the alert does not go to a call centre but to the carer's pager. Both systems can be purchased privately or provided free or with a small fee following assessment by a health professional, such as an OT. There are many different sensors and alarms available, including:

- **Personal alarms** The person wears either a pendant or watch-style alarm. If she falls or feels unwell, she can press the button to raise the alarm.
- **Bed or chair sensors** Pressure mats can be placed under a chair or mattress and set off an alert if someone has got up and not returned within a set time.
- **Door sensors** These detect if someone leaves a room or goes out the front door.
- **Home safety sensors** These include carbon monodioxide, natural gas, and smoke detectors (p.31).

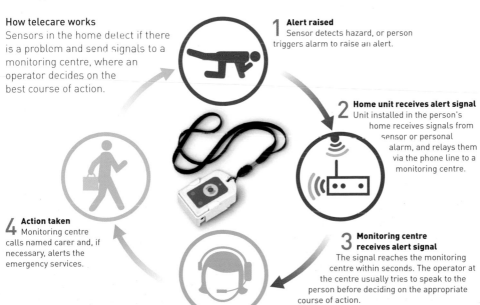

How telecare works
Sensors in the home detect if there is a problem and send signals to a monitoring centre, where an operator decides on the best course of action.

1 Alert raised
Sensor detects hazard, or person triggers alarm to raise an alert.

2 Home unit receives alert signal
Unit installed in the person's home receives signals from sensor or personal alarm, and relays them via the phone line to a monitoring centre.

3 Monitoring centre receives alert signal
The signal reaches the monitoring centre within seconds. The operator at the centre usually tries to speak to the person before deciding on the appropriate course of action.

4 Action taken
Monitoring centre calls named carer and, if necessary, alerts the emergency services.

CHANGED RELATIONSHIPS

It takes time to develop a caring relationship so that you and the person you are caring for can establish a balance of help and independence. Elderly people can be fiercely independent and insist on carrying out their daily routine in their own way, even though it may be clear that they are struggling and may be putting themselves at risk.

Caring for a friend or neighbour

Providing care for a friend or neighbour is very different from caring for a spouse, partner, or relative. The relationship may not be as close and it may feel especially awkward if personal care is necessary. If at any time you are doing more than you really want to, see if you can find others to help, such as the person's family members or social services. Being uncomfortable with the level of care expected may lead to resentment of the person you are caring for, and the relationship may suffer. It is easy for care responsibilities to escalate. You may have started by doing the shopping once a week or taking the person to an occasional hospital appointment. If the person's condition has since deteriorated, you may find that you're now expected to help with feeding, dressing, and bathing.

If caring is taking up more time than you can give, have an honest discussion with the person you are caring for. Explain that you cannot continue providing the same level of care, but that you will help find alternative sources of support. This might be through social services or from local charities or voluntary organizations (p.214).

Caring for your parent

It can be very distressing to care for an elderly and frail parent when that person has always been the one you have relied on. Conversely, it can be very difficult for an elderly parent to be looked after by her child as she may feel guilty about having to rely on you when it is clear that you have your own life's commitments. You need to decide if you feel able to offer your parent full care yourself, or if in fact you would prefer not to be the primary carer. Caring for a relative may help you to grow closer or it may strain the relationship.

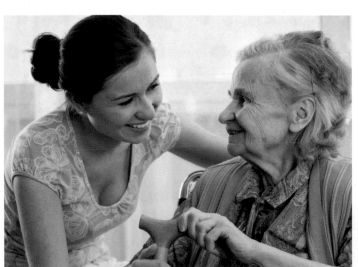

A close bond
Caring for your elderly parent or grandparent can bring you closer together, although you both need to adjust to your changed roles.

Changed roles Even when we are grown up, we tend to think that our parents will always be there for us, providing love and support no matter what. When we realize that a parent now relies on us for care, there may be a sense of loss and bereavement. Equally, a parent who needs care may find it difficult to accept that she is no longer the protector and must now look to her child for help. You may see caring for your parent as a way of repaying her for the care she has given you. However, if you feel there is an expectation that you should take on the role of carer, you may become resentful, which can lead to feelings of guilt (p.21).

Sharing care It may be an advantage to have a care assistant (p.22) do certain tasks. This may be necessary if, as a daughter or son, for instance, you feel you cannot wash and change your father or mother if he or she is becoming incontinent and needs help with personal hygiene. This may not be appropriate or culturally acceptable to you or to your parent.

Some elderly people feel embarrassed to be washed and dressed by someone else, and dignity may be preserved if a son or daughter does not do it. If the care assistant focuses on more intimate care, such as personal hygiene and dressing, it may leave you more time to be involved with mealtimes or activities. This may enable you to create or maintain a more "normal" relationship with your parent.

Caring for your spouse or partner

Becoming your partner's carer changes the nature of your relationship. Where once there was give and take equally between partners, now one partner is providing care and support while the other is likely to become increasingly dependent.

Understanding your feelings You'll probably feel sad because your partner is ill. However, you may also feel angry and resentful because the future you once planned together has been taken away.

When caring for a partner with an illness that affects her mentally, such as Alzheimer's disease, there is the additional emotional burden of the loss of the partner that was. You may feel you no longer recognize your partner as the person you once shared your life with. In this case it is normal to experience feelings of despair, anger, hurt, or bereavement that your partner is not longer able to fulfil the important role she had with you in a former time.

Your sexual relationship Your partner's illness may have had a physical effect so that a sexual relationship becomes difficult. Alternatively, providing intimate care may have caused you to feel that sex might be distasteful or inappropriate. However, sex can be important in a relationship. Try to talk to your partner about your feelings to prevent tensions and feelings of isolation building up. If you find it difficult to talk about this, ask your doctor for a referral to someone who can help.

ALLOWING PERSONAL CHOICE

It may be tempting to rush in and try to do everything because you can see the person is struggling and you are more able.

However, it is important to allow the person to do as much as she can for herself in the way that she wants to. This helps to preserve her skills and abilities. It also preserves her

dignity by enabling her to follow her own routines and live in her chosen way.

It may help you both to sit down and work out together what she does and does not need help with. You can devise either a daily or weekly plan together, which can include a discussion of her worries and abilities.

LOOKING AFTER YOURSELF

Caring can have a much more significant effect on your own health than you realize. Research shows that carers are much more likely to suffer from ill health than those who are not in a caring role.

Your health needs

You may feel that you have no time to care for yourself, or you may be struggling to cope with the burden of care if the condition of the person you look after has deteriorated recently.

However, it is important to make your own health a priority. You will not be able to give your best if you are tired or stressed, and you will find it difficult to carry out your caring tasks if you become ill. A good diet, adequate sleep, exercise, and positive emotional health (p.20) are the mainstays of good overall health.

Professional support

Make sure you tell your own doctor that you are an informal carer so that you will be able to get the advice and support you need. If you have health problems in the future, your doctor will be better able to diagnose and treat you if he or she is already aware of your situation.

Even though your life as a carer is busy, ensure you make time to attend any regular appointments for health tests or screening. Consider asking your doctor for a health checkup, which includes checking your weight, blood pressure, and urine. At this appointment you'll also have the opportunity to discuss any health worries you may have.

In the UK, the local authority has a legal responsibility to help meet the needs of carers, and you are entitled to have a needs assessment (p.211) in much the same way as the person you are looking after is entitled to assessment of her needs (p.12). See your local authority's website for how to apply for a needs assessment (p.216).

Healthy eating

By eating nutritional, balanced meals you'll have more energy to cope with your busy

---

HOW IS CARING AFFECTING YOU?

Caring for someone demands time, energy, and dedication and it can be all too easy to lose sight of your own needs. It is important that you take time periodically to assess what effects being a carer may be having on you.

Questions to ask yourself

- Can you get out alone in order to carry out your personal needs?

- Is your health being negatively affected?

- Is your care role affecting your ability to care for the rest of your family members?

- Is your care role affecting your job?

- Is your care role affecting your financial situation?

Assessing your answers

If you answered "No" to either of the first two questions or "Yes" to any of the last four, then you need to think about how to improve your situation.

Taking action

You can get various kinds of help to make caring easier. Talk to your local authority.

- You may be entitled to a care assistant (p.22) to help you with daily tasks or respite care (p.23) to give you a break from caring.

- Equally important is to ask for more equipment to help make your caring easier or safer.

- Financial help is also available to carers and those they care for (pp.204–213).

day and you'll also be safeguarding your long-term health. You can tailor meals to meet your own nutritional needs as well as those of the person you are caring for. For more information on diet, see pp.44–63.

Getting enough sleep

Not getting adequate sleep contributes greatly to a lack of patience, and also means that your coping mechanisms are less effective, so that you are more likely to become angry, frustrated, and stressed. It is therefore important that you take steps to ensure you don't become overtired.

■ **Regular bedtime** After you have helped the person you are caring for settle into bed, it may be tempting to catch up on tasks or your personal jobs, such as emailing or calling friends. You may find that you're then getting to bed very late. By establishing a routine time for bed, this is less likely to happen.

■ **Daytime naps** If the person has naps during the day, you might be well advised to rest too so that you feel revived enough to easily manage the afternoon and evening care tasks.

■ **Help for disturbed nights** You may find that your nights are being disturbed by the person, for example because she needs frequent trips to the toilet or is suffering from night-time hallucinations (p.107). If you are woken up night after night by such disturbances, it will not be long before you are feeling exhausted. If this is the case it is best to take advice from your doctor as to how best to manage the disturbed nights.

Rest and recovery
A persistent lack of sleep has been associated with raised stress levels. Ensure you get enough rest to allow your body to regenerate.

Making time for exercise

If you are a busy carer, it may be difficult for you to find the time to exercise. If so, try to build your own exercise into the day at the same time you might be encouraging the person you care for to exercise.

■ **Walking** By choosing different routes for a daily walk, you'll not only benefit physically but also emotionally from the opportunities this provides for stimulating fresh conversation. If the person you are caring for cannot walk far, consider finding out about mobility scooters or wheelchairs from your local authority.

■ **Chair and floor exercises** There is a range of good exercises (pp.95–100); some that you can both do, albeit at different levels.

■ **Yoga** This has many benefits, both for people with health problems as well as those who are fit and healthy. It has been shown to greatly improve balance in older people, decreasing the risk of falls.

■ **Swimming** Most public swimming pools offer evening sessions if you manage to have time off then. Or, you may be able to go with the person you are caring for, depending on her level of disability.

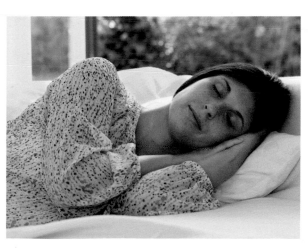

YOUR EMOTIONAL WELLBEING

Although you may be able to manage a positive disposition most days, there are likely to be times when you get quite stressed, and may feel upset, angry, and frustrated. It is very normal to feel stressed when you are coping daily with looking after someone else as well as yourself. There are many tasks to be done each and every day again and again, and you might find yourself feeling moody, sad, resentful, and guilty.

Alleviating stress

It is important to recognize when you are feeling stressed and do something about it. If you ignore your stress, then your daily care tasks will become more difficult to cope with and can negatively affect your own health in the long run.

■ **Minimize social isolation** It is very easy to become so tied up with the all-encompassing role of being a carer that you become isolated before you realize it.

You may be too busy to pick up the phone to your friends, and they may not realize how overwhelmed you might be feeling. Friends may not want to bother you if they think you are too busy, or they may be feeling inadequate themselves because they don't understand the needs of the person you are caring for. They may be frightened of saying the wrong thing or not know how to react if the person has difficult behaviour.

You may be able to cope better if you build into your week some positive actions that will underpin and reinforce your coping ability. Rather than ignoring friends, enlist their help. Set up a rota of people to visit you regularly, perhaps to go for walks or to come for tea or for a drink in the evenings. Talk openly and honestly about the kind of day you have had, or the illness the person

is suffering from so that your friends understand better. Accept help when it is offered. Everyone benefits from more love and support.

■ **Plan your day** Take steps to avoid feeling overwhelmed by your daily round of duties. Making a rough plan for each day can help you feel more in control and less worried about not being able to cope.

Look at the tasks you need to do each day and try to prioritize them. Do they all really need to be done? There may be some, such as ironing, that you can hand over to a friend or family member. Being overtired is a major contributor to stress, so make sure you build in some rest time for you.

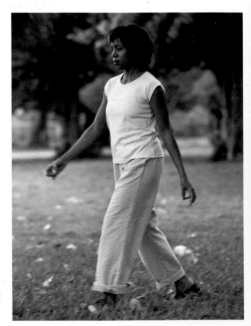

A breath of fresh air
Taking time out for yourself is not as selfish as it may initially feel. By tending to your own needs you will feel more positive and energetic, and be able to offer better care.

■ **Make time for yourself** Give yourself an important, achievable treat each week and do some small but enjoyable things every day. Many people get pleasure from listening to a favourite radio programme, playing a game, taking a long bath with some relaxing aromatherapy oils in the water, playing music, or having the company of a friend.

Inevitably, there are times when a longer break is needed, both from your daily chores and from the person you are caring for. You may feel guilty about wanting a break, but having some time away can allow you to put things into perspective and reduces stress levels. It also enables you to pursue your own interests and hobbies and to retain your sense of self as an independent person. A break will help keep the relationship with the person you are looking after fresh as you will have new experiences to talk about. There are several options for respite care to allow you to have a break (p.23).

Understanding negative feelings

Caring for someone with a long-term disability can be emotionally exhausting, and it is normal to experience a range of negative feelings, which may include:
■ Feelings of inadequacy in your role.
■ Feelings that your relative or friend's suffering is undeserved.
■ Feelings of being trapped into a caring role that you may not have chosen to do.
■ Anger with the person you are caring for.
■ Guilt because you assume that you have no right to feel this way.
■ A sense of loss, or even bereavement, for the once normal and healthy person you knew and loved.

If you can understand why you have these feelings, then you will have gone at least some of the way towards dealing with them. The worst thing you can do is not to acknowledge your feelings. You may be

LOOKING AFTER YOURSELF

There may be times when everything does feel too much and you begin to realize you are feeling depressed. How can you know if you really are depressed and not just overtired?

■ Do you feel inadequate and unable?
■ Are you having difficulty sleeping even when you are not having a disturbed night, or are you waking early?
■ Are you extremely tired most of the time?
■ Are you especially tearful?
■ Are you easily irritated?
■ Do you keep forgetting things and lose concentration easily?
■ Are you forgetting to eat or are you overeating for comfort?

If you have answered "Yes" to some of these questions, then it is time to talk to your own doctor, who might refer you for counselling or possibly prescribe antidepressant medication.

ashamed to talk about them, but if you bottle them up they can become overwhelming. Unrecognized anger, for example, can escalate and lead to irrational judgments and taking out these feelings on the cared for person.

■ **Getting help** If you don't feel able to talk to your friends, consider joining a support group (p.25). Counselling might also be of benefit. This can help you to re-find your own balance while helping you to recognize why you are not coping, and it can show you new ways to approach difficult challenges.

Your doctor or social services should be able to give you further information on counselling and help you to find a counsellor. Before you commit yourself to counselling, meet or speak with the counsellor to find out if he or she makes you feel at ease as you will need to be able to discuss personal details with him or her.

GETTING HELP AND SUPPORT

Caring is a demanding role, and you may need to find someone to help you with day-to-day practical care. Even if you have help, you will occasionally need to have a complete break from caring and either get someone to take over with full-time care or arrange for the person to stay in a residential home while you are away. This is known as respite care.

Care assistants

You can share the caring role with a care assistant. A care assistant can bring more objectivity than you may have been able to, as you will probably have been so closely involved with the person receiving care.

When caring for someone you love, emotions can get in the way and prevent you sometimes from making sensible decisions or caring enough for yourself. It is not possible to be completely detached from the emotional connection of a caring role. An outside care assistant can achieve this while helping you either to give the care or to have a break from it. A care assistant may not have the depth of feeling or the emotional attachment that you have, but he or she will have the correct skills to give the right kind of care.

■ **What does a care assistant do?** A care assistant can give day-to-day practical help like you have been giving. A good care assistant will take note of how you have been providing care, paying attention to how you like the care to be given and how the person likes to be cared for. He or she will also gradually be able to build a relationship with the person.

A care assistant can provide daily care such as washing and dressing, helping with meals, and helping the person to the toilet. He or she can also help with basic housework tasks in the home and will be able to do other tasks with, or for, the person in much the same way as you have been doing. You can let the care assistant know what is most important.

Some care assistants come a couple of times a day if that is enough to care for the person's basic needs. Depending on your needs and that of the person, you may decide you need a carer to stay all day, or even overnight to maintain safety. Some care assistants can move in, and work between five and six days a week. You will have to arrange cover in order for the care assistant to have time off just as you need to have. While you are having a break the

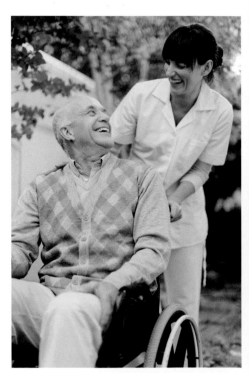

Sharing the load
Not only will use of a care assistant make your life easier, it can also be enlivening for the person to enjoy the company of somebody new.

care assistant can also liaise with some of the other professional people involved, such as the person's doctor or specialist nurse. She can also help the person to take part in recreational activities.

You will want to feel reassured that the care assistant helping you has the correct experience, qualifications, and police checks so that you can feel the person you are caring for is in safe hands. It is equally important to know that he or she is skilled in caring, empathy, and respect for the person he or she will be looking after. This may be more important than qualifications. However, experience is vital if the person will be looking after someone with dementia. Most experienced care assistants are registered with care agencies that help to recruit, train, and vet their staff, taking away some of the worry from you.

An important factor when considering using an outside carer is the cost (p.24). This may be a deciding factor in how often or for how long you use someone.

■ **Finding a care assistant** You can start by contacting your local social services department, who can provide contact details of recommended care agencies. You can also search on the internet, or put an advertisement in your local shops or newspaper. Sometimes people who have been working as cleaners can, if they have the skills, extend their role and do a bit of caring for you, which can give you a short break. The advantage of this is that the person may already know the cleaner and feel comfortable with him or her.

It is always important to check with the person you are caring for as to her opinion about whoever you are thinking of using to help with care. The person needs to feel safe and comfortable with the carer, or the arrangement is not going to work. The care assistant must have the skills and patience to be able to build a relationship no matter how demanding the person may be.

CHOOSING A CARE ASSISTANT

When choosing a care assistant, there are a number of factors to consider.

Assessing suitability
- Are you are able to relate to the person who is going to be helping you with the caring?
- Do you get a good feeling about him or her?
- Is he or she able to be tactful, respectful, and patient?
- Does he or she have a warm and sympathetic approach?
- Does he or she seem to have the ability to relate to the person who needs care?
- Can he or she demonstrate reliability? Did the carer turn up on time?
- Can he or she work the hours or days you need or do you have to make compromises?
- Can he or she demonstrate an understanding of the need to listen to the person enough to promote her dignity and choices?
- Does he or she show an awareness of the need to safeguard a vulnerable person?

Warning
- If using an agency, check that it is properly registered.
- If you are not using an agency, check the care assistant is registered self-employed, is fully insured to do the requisite work, and can provide you with references.

Respite care

There are several options for respite care. Your choice will depend on the needs of the person you are looking after, how long you'll be away, and the cost of the services.

■ **Care at home** Arranging for someone to come into the person's home to look after her while you take a break has the advantage that she remains in familiar surroundings. If you already use a care assistant on a part-time basis, then the ideal solution is for that person to extend his or her hours and provide full-time care for a short period. If you don't already have a care assistant, ask the local authority for their recommended care agencies.

» GETTING HELP AND SUPPORT

Alternatively, you could find a carer through personal recommendation or through local advertisements. Make sure that the person you choose is registered self-employed and is fully insured to do the requisite work.

- **Day centre care** The person you are looking after can go to a day centre or participate in activities away from home, enabling you to have full or part days away from caring. Services provided vary, but many include occupational therapy, such as art, keep fit, and craft work.
- **Residential care** In this type of care, the person being cared for stays for a short time in a residential or nursing home.
- **Respite holiday** A number of different organizations arrange holidays for people with disabilities or special needs, making it possible for the person you are looking after to have a holiday while you have a break. You can also go away together.

Funding for care

Funding for a care assistant is based on a community care assessment (p.12). Some local authorities will also offer respite care based on a community care assessment, but others will base their decision on a carer's needs assessment (p.211). Therefore, it's best for both you and the person you are looking after to be assessed individually. The type and amount of care offered will depend on the results of the assessments and varies in different parts of the country. The person you are caring for may also be entitled to an Attendance Allowance (p.206)

Instead of offering services directly, local authorities may give you the choice of a direct payment to you or the person you are looking after. This is a sum of money that can be used to employ staff or to buy services from a voluntary or private agency. It can also be used to help cover the cost of respite care. It enables you to fund the replacement care in whatever way you like and to choose how you want to spend your time off.

If you are unable to get funding from local authorities for the care you need, there are many voluntary organizations, holiday organizations, and charities that can help (p.214).

Going on holiday together

You may want to go on holiday with the person you are caring for. With a little forward planning, this is perfectly possible. There are several organizations that cater for elderly and disabled people (p.216). Before you book a holiday, talk to the tour operator to make sure that the holiday

ASKING FRIENDS AND FAMILY FOR HELP

Friends and family are often willing to offer help so that you can take a break from caring.

This arrangement can have several advantages over more formal respite care.

- The person will feel more at ease being looked after by someone she knows.
- You will feel more comfortable leaving the person in a safe and familiar pair of hands.

- Someone who knows the person may be more familiar with her routine and her likes and dislikes.

- You'll avoid the bureaucracy and cost of arranging for respite care.

Do remember, however, that family and friends may find caring over a continuous period more stressful than anticipated and also may not be available to give you a break when you need it.

centre can cater for the needs of the person you are looking after. For example, if the person has limited mobility, ask whether there are ground-floor rooms, and lifts or stair lifts. Ask about facilities in the bathroom, such as handrails and hoists, and whether beds are adjustable. If the person needs medical care, it's important that suitable trained staff are available.

Before you book a holiday, make sure the person you are caring for can get travel insurance that covers her for health problems that may occur while on holiday. When taking out insurance, any disabilities or illness must be declared, or the insurance is not valid.

Getting there The travel company may be able to arrange for transport to and from stations and airports. Alternatively, seek assistance from a local voluntary organization. Most rail companies will offer help if they are told ahead of time to expect a disabled passenger, and airlines also must offer a person assistance with getting on and off aeroplanes.

Support groups

Getting together with others who share your experiences as a carer can help you to feel less isolated and is a good way to get all sorts of useful information. Some types of support group, such as Macmillan Cancer support, deal with a particular condition. Others are there to give support to the carer, such as Carer's UK, Crossroads Care, and the Princess Royal Trust for Carers. Many of these groups have local branches around the country. Local councils also often run local support

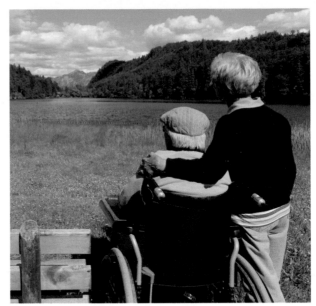

Take a break
Enjoying a holiday with the person you are looking after is a good way of injecting new life into your routine together.

groups. Contact your local social services department for details.

■ **Benefits of support groups** Joining a support group is a great way to make new friends who understand exactly what you are going through. Others who have had the same problems as you will not only be able to offer you kindness and sympathy, but also practical tips. Other benefits of support groups may include: access to up-to date information about your benefits and rights as a carer; social activities; and specific training, such as learning how to move someone without damaging your back. The precise services offered will vary from group to group.

■ **Starting a support group** If you can't find a group near you that suits your needs, think about setting one up. You'll need to consider your aim, how you'll advertise the group, and where you will hold meetings.

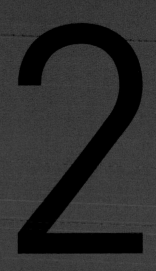

2

MAKING CHANGES
TO THE HOME

■ WHERE TO GET ADVICE AND HELP ■ GENERAL ADAPTATIONS
■ HOME SAFETY AND SECURITY ■ EXTERNAL ACCESS
■ HALLWAYS AND STAIRS ■ SITTING ROOM ■ KITCHEN
■ BEDROOM ■ BATHROOM

WHERE TO GET ADVICE AND HELP

When you think about how to adapt a home to suit a person's particular needs, it is important to consider costs, aesthetics, the impact of the adaptation on the home, and how it may affect other household members. Before considering any adaptations that may be required, you will need to decide where the person you are caring for will be living. Would he be better off staying in his own home or could moving in with you be more practical, especially if he requires a higher level of care. You need to be realistic and, in some cases, care in a care home may be the best option.

Rushing into decisions can be costly both in monetary and emotional terms, so consider changes carefully and seek professional advice.

The level of changes to the home

The extent of adaptations and changes carried out in the home will depend on the circumstances of the person you are caring for. If you are caring for someone who is convalescing for a short period of time after an illness, you will want to avoid making expensive changes and look for practical, low-cost adaptations. For example, relocating a bed to the sitting room may not be an ideal long-term solution, but may be practical if needed for just a few weeks to avoid going up and down stairs. If specialist equipment is needed for a short period of time, check whether you might be able to borrow or rent this from a voluntary organization. .

Getting professional advice

Before making any adaptations to the home, it's advisable to get professional advice and help. The best source for this will usually be an occupational therapist. Occupational therapists are health professionals who specialize in enabling people with limited mobility, illness, or other special needs to maintain their maximum level of independence in the home. Part of their job is to help people re-learn or adapt skills so that they can carry out everyday tasks and activities. They also give advice on equipment and adaptations to the home, and can make the necessary arrangements for the adaptations to be carried out.

In the UK, occupational therapists are employed mainly in the NHS and by local authorities and social services, and some are

Talking it through
An occupational therapist will explain to you what adaptations can be carried out to best meet the needs of the person you care for.

Assessing requirements

An occupational therapist can assess whether the width of doorways is sufficient to enable a wheelchair user to move about the house easily. If she determines that widening door frames would be helpful, she can then arrange for this to be carried out.

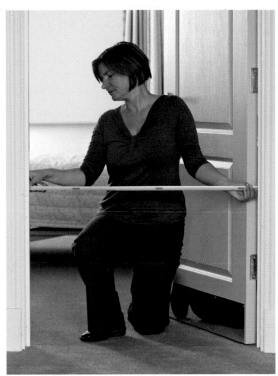

in private practice. They are usually accessed through a doctor, social services, or as an in-patient in hospital. Some UK health authorities have a self-referral system; if the person in your care wishes to self-refer, check with your doctor if this option is available locally.

Before you meet the therapist, it's worth listing all the areas where you feel you and the person you are caring for need help. For example, does he have difficulty accessing toilet facilities because he cannot easily climb stairs, or is answering the door a problem because he finds it difficult to get up from a chair?

Funding for home adaptations

In the UK, whether or not you receive funding for home adaptations is dependent on whether a home is privately owned or rented, council owned, or rented through a housing association (p.214).

If you are eligible for funding, some assessments can be "fast-tracked", which means that a full assessment by a medical professional isn't needed before carrying out work. This may be the case if a change is fairly straightforward and the individual's needs are not complex. He may have been assessed already for a disability allowance (p.207) and have general mobility requirements. A fast-track adaptation may be minor, such as fitting a holding rail, or more major, such as removing a bath to fit a level-access shower.

BUYING EQUIPMENT

There is a vast array of equipment and gadgets designed to help people with particular needs carry out everyday tasks. Items are advertised in newspapers, magazines, on television, and are sold in supermarkets. It can be confusing to know exactly what you need to purchase, and costly if you invest in equipment that turns out to be inappropriate or faulty. To make the right decisions and keep cost down:

■ Research what's available before buying.

■ See if you can try out an item before deciding whether to buy. Check with your local provider what services they offer.

■ In the UK, you can claim VAT exemption. All equipment designed for people with disabilities is exempt from VAT. This must be claimed before purchase; no doctor's letter is required. General retailers who stock furniture may not offer this service, so it is important to check first. Some stockists have VAT exemption forms with their order form.

GENERAL ADAPTATIONS

Some simple changes to the home can make it easier and safer for a person with limited mobility to get around and maintain his independence. If the person you are looking after is elderly, bear in mind, too, that he may be more sensitive to the cold, so it is vitally important that heating is adequate and can be quickly and easily adjusted if the temperature falls.

Suitable flooring

Check the suitability of flooring throughout the home and whether it needs replacing or adapting. Loose rugs and mats can be attractive and protect floors, but are also an obvious tripping hazard. Remove them, fix them securely to the floor with double-sided tape, or invest in non-slip matting. A thick carpet stops heat escaping, but it can be difficult to push wheeled walking frames or wheelchairs over. Linoleum or vinyl flooring is smooth and easy to walk on, but can be cold on top of concrete floors. Tiles are also cold and can be uneven. The advantage of smooth floors is that they are easily cleaned and hard-wearing; however, wheeled walking frames and trolleys can "run away" with the person on smooth surfaces if his walking is unsteady. Low-pile washable carpets or non-slip matting may be preferable.

The right temperature

If the person is elderly, he may need to have heating on all day in the colder months. You could consider energy-efficient portable heaters that release heat over a long period of time. These keep rooms at a constant temperature and avoid overheating.

In hot weather, a portable fan is useful. Look for one that has different settings and that rotates so that air is circulated.

Taps, sockets, and knobs

Turning taps on and off can be tricky for those with a poor grip. Ideally, change taps to lever taps or fit easy-to-grip tap turners, which also reduce the risk of dripping. Raised sockets and plug pulls avoid the need to bend down or reach into corners; and key turners and lever-style handles instead of door knobs make access easier.

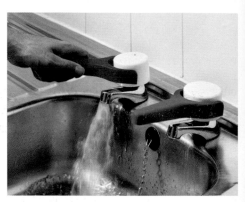

Tap attachments
Colour-coded adjustable tap turners fitted onto taps are easy to grip, making turning taps on and off simple and avoiding wasteful drips.

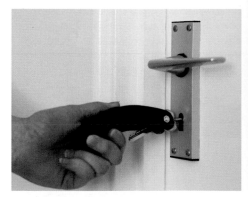

Key turner
Designed to mould around a key, this chunky key holder has an easy-to-hold handle to aid those with a weak grip.

HOME SAFETY AND SECURITY

Reducing the likelihood of any major incident in the home is a priority as a carer, especially if the person being cared for has visual or hearing problems, poor mobility, or is confused, all of which make it harder to recognize risks. There have been vast technological improvements in safety and security products over the last few years, and many are now quite commonplace. Products may be purchased privately or provided, sometimes free of charge or with a small rental fee, following assessment by a health professional such as an occupational therapist. Some safety products, including certain sensors and alarms, are telecare products (p.15): they connect to a monitoring centre and send an alert automatically if a risk is detected.

Safety in the home

Products that are available as part of the telecare system include carbon monoxide and natural gas sensors, smoke detectors, and temperature control sensors. If a danger from gas or smoke is detected, or the temperature falls too low, they sound an alarm or provide a visual cue in the home, while also alerting a monitoring centre. There are also stand-alone safety devices such as a bath plug that detects if the water temperature is too high and also releases excess water to prevent overflow.

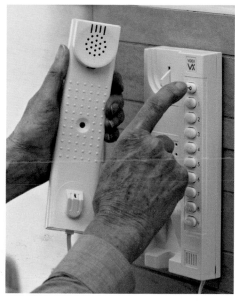

Using an intercom
A home intercom system gives peace of mind. Wall mounted or wireless, these enable a two-way conversation with visitors at the door.

Ensuring security

Key "safes" can be fitted outside the front door to allow access for care staff and family without the need for the person to open the door themselves. Devices such as wireless intercoms and entry systems are also useful, and phone adaptations can be carried out, which provide a built-in alarm/emergency call system.

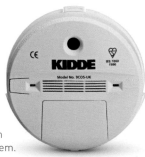

Carbon monoxide sensor
Simple to fit and widely available, carbon monoxide sensors are an essential safety feature in the home. Ensure you choose one with an audible alarm system.

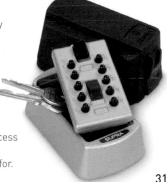

Key safe
A coded key safe with a spare key can be fixed to an outside wall, giving the carer instant access to the home of the person being cared for.

EXTERNAL ACCESS

Often, one of the first adaptations to be carried out to the home is external, ensuring that the person can get in and out of the house safely. Outside changes can include adapting pathways, improving lighting, and ensuring easy accessibility.

Adapting outside steps

If the person finds it difficult to get up and down outside steps, a simple handrail may be all that is needed. If more support is necessary, a wall-to-ground handrail on either one or both sides of the steps may be required. If steps are uneven or the tread is too narrow, you may need to consider carrying out more major adaptations to rebuild or lower steps.

If a person is dependent on a wheelchair, you will need to consider a ramp to aid access. For single steps, you can often use a simple portable ramp, which can be put in place only when needed. However, if there are several steps, you may need to look into installing a permanent ramp system. If this is the case, get professional advice, as there are many considerations, including the width, gradient, and length. For areas where a ramp will not fit or the

rise is too great for a ramp to make economic sense (usually anything over 76cm/30in), you may need to think about installing a wheelchair lift.

Making pathways safe

Assess the condition of outside paths to check whether they are slippery or uneven, and whether they need widening for a wheelchair. Ideally, paths should be level, or just gently sloping. Gravel paths are tricky for wheelchairs to negotiate, so it's best to keep surfaces smooth. Make sure that paths are well lit, and that access to a car in the driveway or to the road is safe. Check, too, that paving stones are even and that vegetation isn't obscuring the path. If there is no off-road parking, find out from the local authority whether the person is eligible for a disabled parking bay.

If the property has an entrance gate, check whether this is wide enough to accommodate a wheelchair if necessary.

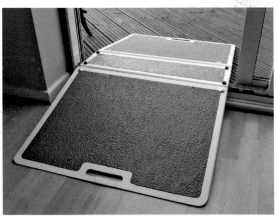

Portable ramps
A non-slip, lightweight portable ramp provides smooth wheelchair access over raised doorways. Choose a longer ramp to reduce the gradient and ensure ease of use.

HALLWAYS AND STAIRS

Inside the home, some of the first areas to look at are the hallway and stairs. It's important that the person you are caring for is able to move around the house with ease as far as possible, so that he can enjoy maximum independence.

Safe hallways

Hallways are often dark with little natural lighting. If this is the case, it is important to ensure that the hallway has good artificial lighting with easily accessed switches. Raised sockets, large switches, and one-touch timer lights or motion sensor lights are all helpful.

Keep hallways de-cluttered, too. Make sure the floor surface is safe, removing or securing any loose mats and rugs, which are a common cause of falls, and check there are no trailing telephone cables that can be tripped over.

Using the stairs

Stairs are one of the most obvious risks for a person with reduced mobility (p.80). A downstairs toilet is ideal to reduce the need to go up and down the stairs throughout the day. Plan, too, what the person you are caring for might need during the course of a day, such as spare clothes and books, so that he can remain on one level until bedtime. If the person needs to use a walking aid, it is useful to have one upstairs and to keep a separate one downstairs so that he doesn't need to carry it up and down or go without.

Extra handrails or banisters may be required to improve stair safety. Make sure they are wide enough to grasp easily. Bear in mind that using two handrails is much easier and safer than one, especially if a staircase is curved and has a narrow tread as it turns.

Installing a stair lift

You may need to think about installing a stair lift if a person is unable to negotiate the stairs and there is no downstairs access to a toilet or bedroom. The type of stair lift will depend on whether the stairs are straight or curved, and whether there is more than one flight. There also needs to be sufficient access at the bottom and top for getting on and off safely. Other considerations include whether the person will be able to manage the controls independently, and if other household members can negotiate their way past the stair lift when it's not in use.

A stair lift is a considerable investment, so compare prices, including the cost of warranties and maintenance contracts, and seek advice on suitable models.

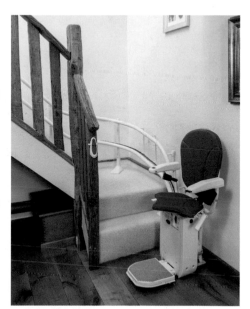

Stair lift
For someone with limited mobility who needs to access facilities on more than one level, a stair lift can offer the perfect solution.

SITTING ROOM

This is often the room where the person being cared for spends most of his time during the day, so it's important to ensure it is a safe and pleasant environment. When reviewing the sitting room, think about heating sources, lighting, and whether the person has easy access to the telephone, television controls, and the radio.

One of the most important things to consider is seating, which should be comfortable, supportive, and accessible. You also need to think about the position of seating: place it in the best position in the room, ideally near a window so the person has a view out, although not in direct sunlight or near draughts.

General adaptations to the sitting room

There are several factors to consider when assessing the safety and suitability of the sitting room.

First, assess floor coverings. Loose mats or thick hearth rugs can provide comfort and warmth, as well as being decorative, but can also be a tripping hazard. Either secure them or remove them altogether.

If there is an open fire in the room, think about the associated risks. Ensure there is a fire guard in place, that fires are put out properly after use, and that the chimney is maintained. Alternatively, consider other heating sources. If central heating hasn't been installed, check whether a grant is available to switch to central heating.

Raised sockets and plug-pulling devices make it easier to switch off electric fires and televisions. Gas controls on fires can be converted to easy-to-turn knobs, and carbon monoxide sensors are essential.

If the person being cared for has very limited mobility, you may want to consider remote control curtains and lights to enable him to control his environment.

Assessing seating

Bad seating can lead to poor sitting posture, which can in turn exacerbate or lead to other problems, such as backache.

HOW TO MEASURE FOR A CHAIR

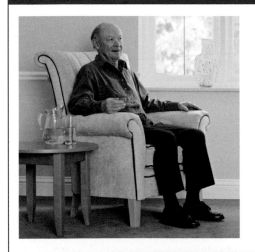

If you are helping the person you are caring for to purchase a new chair, you need to ensure that it is supportive and that its dimensions will allow him to get in and out with ease.

- The chair should be wide enough to allow the person's hands to slide down easily either side of the hips.

- The depth of the seat should be about 3–5cm (1–2in) short of knee length to stop the chair digging into the back of the knee or encouraging a slumped posture.

- The seat should be at last 4–5cm (1½–2in) higher than the knee-to-floor length, although not so high that the person has trouble putting his feet flat on the floor.

- A footstool can be useful if a higher seat is needed to make standing easier.

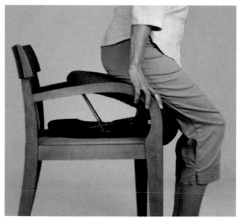

Ejector spring cushion
Either manual or battery operated, a spring cushion tilts at an angle to assist getting out of a chair. It should only be used on chairs with arms.

Seating needs to provide support while also being comfortable, and the person should be able to get in and out of a chair with ease. Sometimes, seating can meet certain criteria but be unsuitable in another area. For example, a person may have a favourite chair that he finds comfortable but which is difficult to get up from.

There are several common problems with seating. A sagging base on a chair contributes to poor sitting posture. People sometimes try to solve this problem by using an extra cushion, but this may not be the same size as the base and can be unstable. If the chair seat is too long, the person has to slide forwards into a slumped position to get his feet on the floor, making it difficult to get up and out of the chair. Sometimes the chair itself is too low, which also makes it difficult to get out of it.

Seating solutions

There are various adaptations that can be carried out to help ensure that seating is comfortable and supportive.
■ A chair raiser can be placed under the

castors or legs to raise the chair 5cm (2in) or more. The raise is similar to that used to raise up a bed (p.39).
■ A firm base cushion, measured to fit the chair snugly, can be added. This raises the base of the seat and is especially suitable for those who have sufficient mobility and strength in their legs, so that they don't need to push up from the chair arms to get out of the chair.
■ An ejector spring cushion (left) can be used. This helps the person to rise gently from the chair as his weight is lifted off the cushion. The chair needs to have proper arm rests for the person to hold on to as the seat rises.

Alternatively, you may want to consider purchasing a new chair to meet the specific requirements of the person you are caring for. This could be:
■ An ordinary chair that fits well (see panel, opposite) and meets the criteria for support and comfort. A high-backed chair is particularly suitable, as this provides good back support.
■ A manual or electric riser recliner chair (below).

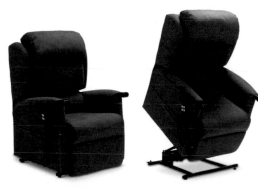

Electric riser recliner chairs
Specifically designed for those with limited mobility, these chairs recline or gently bring the sitter to his feet at the touch of a button.

KITCHEN

The degree of adaptation required in the kitchen will depend on the level of mobility of the person you are caring for. If he is a wheelchair user and would like to use the kitchen independently, then major adaptations will be necessary. Simpler interventions and equipment can be introduced to make meal preparation easier and safer for a person with reduced dexterity and/or movement. Maintaining independence in the kitchen is beneficial for you both, easing the burden on you and increasing the person's sense of self-worth.

Major adaptations

There are several adaptations that can be made in the kitchen for wheelchair users. These include installing wheelchair accessible sinks that are low, and have space underneath for the wheelchair, and accessible cupboards and work surfaces. Work surfaces can be lowered in general, or pull-out surfaces can be installed at the correct level for the wheelchair user. As with all wheelchair access, doorways may need widening and the flooring should be level and smooth.

Minor adaptations

Some simple commonsense changes can make items accessible so that the need for bending and stretching is reduced. Place commonly used items on work surfaces or in easy-to-reach cupboards, and avoid using low or high shelves. A perching stool is helpful if the person has difficulty standing for long periods of time to prepare food, and a kitchen walking trolley or a caddy that attaches to a walking frame is essential if he needs a walking support to carry items across the room.

If space permits, have a table and chair in the kitchen for eating, so that hot food and drinks or heavy trays don't have to be carried from one room to another.

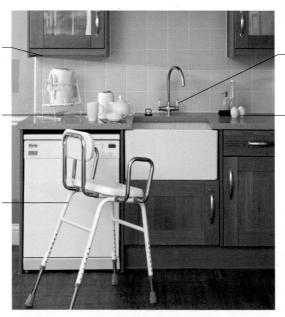

Install strip lighting under cupboards to maximize visibility

Keep separate items needed for specific tasks, such as making tea, in one place

A lightweight, portable chair (perching stool) that can be drawn up to a work surface helps those with less stamina to spend time on tasks such as food preparation

Lever-type taps are easier to use for people with a poor grip

Store frequently used items on work surfaces or in accessible drawers or cupboards

An accessible kitchen
Adapting and arranging the kitchen to ensure ease of use helps to maintain independence. Even small changes can make a significant difference.

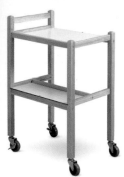

Kitchen trolley
An easy-to-manoeuvre kitchen trolley reduces the need for lifting and carrying around the kitchen, and is useful for transporting hot dishes to the table.

Visual aids and reminders
If the person has poor vision and/or memory problems, there are several measures that can be taken to help ensure he is able to use the kitchen safely and easily. Bright markers on the microwave and cooker can highlight commonly used cooking times. A cooker "guard" safety device can be connected to the cooker, which turns it off automatically if it is left on too long, and a hob guard can protect the visually impaired from accidentally knocking hot pans.

You can also purchase liquid-level indicators, which are units placed on the side of a cup that vibrate or beep when the cup is nearly full. There are special safety overflow plugs that can be placed in the kitchen sink to help reduce the risk of flooding if a tap is left on.

KITCHEN EQUIPMENT

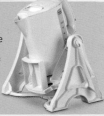

Kettle tipper
The kettle is placed in a tipper device to avoid the need for heavy lifting, in turn reducing the risk of scalds and burns.

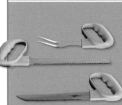

Ergonomic food preparation knives
An adapted handle keeps the wrist in a neutral position, so less strength is needed to chop.

"One touch" jar and tin opener
Battery-operated or electric tin openers are easier to manage than manual ones for those with limited dexterity.

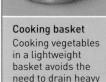

Saucepans
Two-handled saucepans and ones with angled handles are easier to hold and handle while cooking.

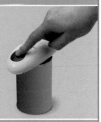

Cooking basket
Cooking vegetables in a lightweight basket avoids the need to drain heavy pans of hot water.

Bread buttering/spike board
Spikes secure food and raised edges hold bread in place for buttering. These are useful for those who can use only one hand.

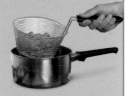

BEDROOM

The person you are caring for may need to spend a considerable amount of time in the bedroom, so it's important that it is comfortable, with sufficient space around the bed to allow a carer to assist if needed. You need to assess the person's mobility for getting in and out of bed, and ensure good access from the bedroom to the toilet.

General adaptations to the bedroom

It's important that lighting controls can be reached easily while in bed. Place a light (an angled one is good for reading) beside the bed, ideally on a bedside table, as well as a torch in case of an emergency. Night-lights and motion sensor lights that come on automatically when they sense movement are useful, too. A telephone should be within easy reach, and a clock clearly visible; digital clocks are often easier to read. Remove, or secure, loose-lying mats and any general clutter, and ensure there is a clear passageway from the bedside to the door and the toilet. If the person has a walking frame or wheelchair, the door frame needs to be wide enough to accommodate this.

A sturdy table tray or cantilever table that can be drawn in over the bed is useful for eating meals and snacks in bed, and for placing books and magazines on. Other useful reading aids include a reading stand that facilitates reading while lying or sitting in bed, and manual or electric page turners to assist those with limited dexterity.

If space is available, place an upright chair next to the bed, for the person to sit on when he wishes during the day and for visitors to use.

If a toilet aid such as a commode (p.136) is required, this will also need to be kept close to the bed.

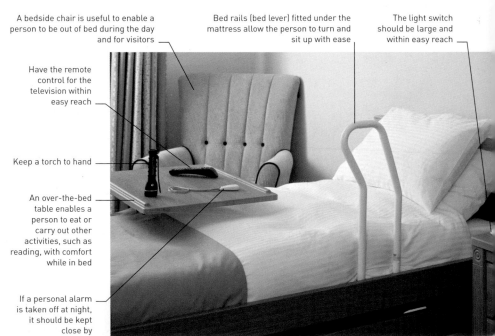

A bedside chair is useful to enable a person to be out of bed during the day and for visitors

Bed rails (bed lever) fitted under the mattress allow the person to turn and sit up with ease

The light switch should be large and within easy reach

Have the remote control for the television within easy reach

Keep a torch to hand

An over-the-bed table enables a person to eat or carry out other activities, such as reading, with comfort while in bed

If a personal alarm is taken off at night, it should be kept close by

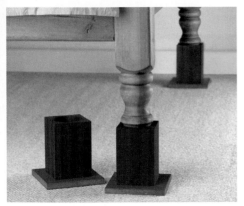

Bed raisers

Individual bed raisers are a quick, convenient way to raise the height of the bed, making it easier to get on and off the bed.

Adapting the bed

Various adaptations and items can be used to help a person with reduced mobility get in and out of bed. If the bed is fairly low, it can be hard for the person being cared for to get in and out independently and for you to assist him. If this is the case, you may need to use bed raisers (above). Some special adjustable beds (p.108) can be lowered to make getting in or out easier.

There are also aids called leg lifters that help a person lift his legs back onto the bed. An electronic leg lifter consists of a small platform that fits onto the side of an adjustable bed. A manual leg lifter is a reinforced strap with a loop through which a person places his foot. Short bed rails, also called a bed lever, can be fitted under the mattress and positioned near the head of the bed to help with turning and levering up (p.114 shows how a bed lever is used). Grab rails on the wall or swing-out bed rails or poles can assist with standing once a person is out of bed.

Devices referred to as "monkey" poles and bed ladders, which allow a person to hold onto a bar, or support and pull himself upright in bed, are available, although these are used less frequently now because they can lead to shoulder injuries.

If a person's mobility is severely limited, a hoist (p.88) can be used to lift him into or out of bed.

Sitting up in bed

If a person needs to spend extended periods of time in bed, it is worth investing in aids to help him sit up comfortably and supported. Adjustable back rests, wedges, and V-shaped pillows (p.110) are available.

Electronic mattress elevators that raise the pillow end are also available. Or, for long-term situations, you may want to consider investing in an electric adjustable bed, which adapts the position of the head and foot ends separately to suit the needs of the individual.

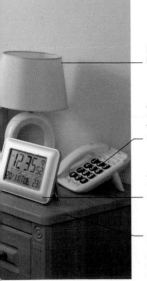

Ensure lighting is adequate

A bedside phone is useful. Adapted phones with large numbers are easy to use

A digital clock is often easier to read than an analogue one

An easy-to-reach bedside table provides a useful surface; ensure it is level with the pillow height

The right environment

Ensuring that everyday items are close to hand when in bed can avoid frustration and isolation, and ensure the person is sufficiently stimulated.

BATHROOM

Bathrooms are frequently problematic for people with reduced mobility. They are often small with restricted turning areas, can be slippery, and baths are difficult to get out of. Bathrooms are also used during the day and the night. There are various adaptations and equipment that help to make bathrooms more user-friendly.

Shower units

An accessible shower is often the best solution for a person with reduced mobility. Standard shower units can be difficult to get into, as they have a step to negotiate. A portable non-slip step makes access easier, and handrails inside the shower aid balance. Free-standing shower stools or wall-mounted ones that flip up out of the way are useful if the person has poor balance or can stand for only limited periods of time.

Over-bath showers can be difficult to access. A bath-board and seat (opposite) can help the person to swing his legs into the bath, then either sit or stand to shower. A wall-mounted handrail helps balance. If the bath has a glass shower panel, the board may not fit across, and a high bath seat may be the only other option. Level-access showers are ideal and allow easy wheelchair access. These usually have rails and wall-mounted seats, and

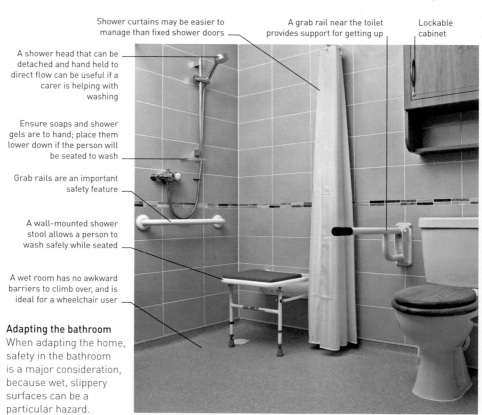

Shower curtains may be easier to manage than fixed shower doors

A grab rail near the toilet provides support for getting up

Lockable cabinet

A shower head that can be detached and hand held to direct flow can be useful if a carer is helping with washing

Ensure soaps and shower gels are to hand; place them lower down if the person will be seated to wash

Grab rails are an important safety feature

A wall-mounted shower stool allows a person to wash safely while seated

A wet room has no awkward barriers to climb over, and is ideal for a wheelchair user

Adapting the bathroom
When adapting the home, safety in the bathroom is a major consideration, because wet, slippery surfaces can be a particular hazard.

come with half-height doors and a curtain, allowing the carer to help with washing without getting soaked themselves.

Wet rooms have no boundary between the shower and the rest of the room, allowing full wheelchair access and space to manoeuvre.

Using the bath

Getting in and out of a bath can be challenging. While the ideal is to replace the bath with a shower unit (unless there is a medical reason for bathing, such as a skin condition that requires immersion in water), there are ways to make baths accessible.

A bath-board and attached seat can be fitted across the top of the bath. However, this requires arm and knee strength to get up and down. Wall rails next to the bath or a grab bar on the side of the bath can help. A battery-operated bath lift enables the person to be lowered further down into the bath. A chair sits in the bath and raises and

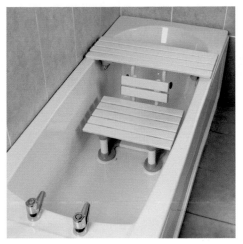

Bath-board
Removable bath-boards that sit across the top of the bath are available in a range of sizes and provide a seated platform to access the bath.

lowers the person by the touch of a button. Users need to be able to lift their legs over the bath. If this is difficult, a swivel bather, which is a floor-fixed chair hoist that swings over the bath, may be preferable.

For comfort, waterproof cushions for sitting on or leaning against are available.

Adapting the toilet

Using the toilet can be difficult for those with reduced mobility and/or dexterity. The following adaptations can help:
- A raised toilet seat (p.134) that clips on to the bowl (the seat and lid are lifted up) makes it easier to get on and off the toilet.
- A toilet frame (p.135) with or without a combined seat provides support.
- Grab rails or flip-down wall rails can be fitted on the wall, or rails can be fixed to the floor.
- A toilet system with integrated washing and drying facilities can be installed for those with limited use of their hands.

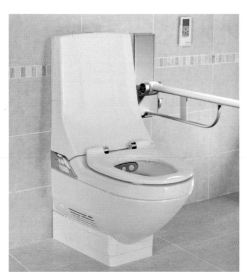

All-in-one toilet
A toilet system that combines an automatic flushing system with a washing and drying facility can help people to use the toilet independently.

3

DIET AND HEALTH

■ EATING WELL ■ MONITORING WEIGHT ■ SPOTTING MALNUTRITION
■ SWALLOWING AND EATING DIFFICULTIES ■ SPECIAL DIETARY NEEDS
■ WHEN FOOD IS NOT ENOUGH ■ THE IMPORTANCE OF MEALTIMES
■ PUTTING EATING WELL INTO PRACTICE
■ FOOD HYGIENE AND FOOD SAFETY

EATING WELL

Eating well means taking in the right amount of energy (calories) and nutrients to enable the body to carry out its normal daily processes as well as to guard against, or recover from, illness or damage.

Importance of eating well

A poor diet can be severely detrimental to health, leading to malnutrition, which has a range of damaging effects (p.46), including poor recovery from illness or surgery. However, many people remain unsure of the amounts and types of food they need to ensure their daily energy and nutritional needs are met. A poor diet also increases the risk of long-term diseases, such as heart disease, high blood pressure, cancer, osteoporosis, obesity, and diabetes.

Food groups

The five main food groups should be eaten in the proportions represented below, with foods in the larger panels forming the greatest part of the diet. The total amount of food needed depends on body size, age, and activity levels.

Components of a healthy diet

The key nutrients needed by the body are fats, carbohydrates (starchy foods), dietary fibre, and minerals. In order to obtain what the body needs requires a diet that is rich in fruits, vegetables, and starchy foods, such as bread or rice; moderate amounts of dairy products, meat, fish, eggs, and other sources of protein, such as pulses and beans; and limited amounts of foods that are high in fat and/or sugar. The two main types of fat found in food are saturated fats – those mainly present in animal products – and unsaturated fats including monounsaturates, which help to reduce cholesterol. Where possible, saturated fats should be replaced with monounsaturates, such as olive oil, rapeseed oil, or soybean oil. The amount of salt in the diet should be small, with alcohol drunk only in moderation. While this nutritional advice aims to promote good health for the general population, much of it remains equally important as a

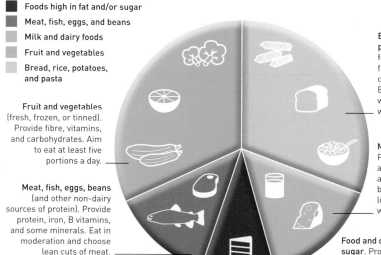

- ■ Foods high in fat and/or sugar
- ■ Meat, fish, eggs, and beans
- ■ Milk and dairy foods
- ■ Fruit and vegetables
- ■ Bread, rice, potatoes, and pasta

Fruit and vegetables (fresh, frozen, or tinned). Provide fibre, vitamins, and carbohydrates. Aim to eat at least five portions a day.

Meat, fish, eggs, beans (and other non-dairy sources of protein). Provide protein, iron, B vitamins, and some minerals. Eat in moderation and choose lean cuts of meat.

Bread, rice, potatoes, and pasta (and other starchy foods). Provide dietary fibre, minerals, including calcium and iron, and B vitamins. Choose wholegrain varieties when possible.

Milk and dairy foods. Provide protein, calcium, and certain vitamins, such as B12, A, and D. Tend to be high in fat, so choose low-fat alternatives where possible.

Food and drink high in fat and/or sugar. Provide energy but intake should be limited – have low-fat alternatives where possible.

person ages or comes to require care. However, it is important to remember that in certain circumstances some people may need to eat a more nutrient-dense diet.

Individual energy and nutrient needs

These are determined by a person's age, gender, body size, the amount of activity she does, and her current state of health. Everyone has different needs, but there are good estimates of average portions for people of different ages and genders that help when it comes to planning the person's meals and assessing whether she is eating enough. It is a good idea to eat well throughout the day to maintain energy levels (p.60).

Who is at nutritional risk?

An imbalanced diet is the key reason for poor nutritional health and can be caused by a number of factors, including poor appetite, a reduced choice of foods, pain or difficulty eating, or difficulties with shopping, cooking, or preparing food (below). Many of these factors tend to be more common in older people, and they are therefore likely to be at the greatest risk. It is well established that malnutrition is common among older people, whether they are living in their own homes or have moved into residential care.

Factors associated with poor nutritional health

An individual's ability or motivation to eat well can be negatively affected for a variety of reasons. It is important to be aware of any of the following situations arising, and take steps to ensure that the person you are looking after does not enter a spiral of poor eating habits as a result.

■ A person who is inactive, or bedbound, or who rarely goes outside, is likely to have smaller than average energy needs. This can make it hard to eat food in sufficient

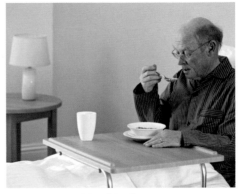

Maintaining nutritional intake
Being confined to bed reduces the appetite, so concentrated, nutrient-rich food that is easy to eat, such as soup, helps maintain nutrient levels.

quantities to consume all the nutrients required. Not going outside also risks developing a vitamin D deficiency (p.47).
■ A person may have a small appetite if she is ill, or if she is living alone.
■ If a person has mouth, swallowing, or chewing problems, she may find eating difficult and may avoid some foods or even avoid meals altogether.
■ Some medicines have side effects, such as drowsiness, nausea, a metallic taste in the mouth, dryness in the mouth, or constipation, which may then impact on a person's food choices or eating pattern.
■ A person with poor sight, hearing, or taste may find mealtimes more difficult.
■ A person suffering from depression or any other psychological problem may be less motivated to eat well, or she may suffer from food anxieties.
■ A person who has communication problems may not like what is offered or may want it at a different temperature or in a different format, but be unable to say so.
■ If a person has a long-term condition, is recovering from illness or surgery, or has a longstanding disability, she might be at risk of malnutrition and so may be in need of a more nutrient-dense diet.

» EATING WELL

Effects of poor diet

If a person does not eat enough food, or if she eats too much of it, or even if she eats a reasonable quantity but it does not contain a good balance of nutrients, she is at risk of malnutrition. Malnutrition can contribute directly to a number of conditions and disorders, including:

- An increased risk of infection.
- Poor or slow wound healing.

NUTRIENTS LIKELY TO BE IN SHORT SUPPLY

NUTRIENT	FUNCTION WITHIN THE BODY	GOOD SOURCES
Vitamin C	■ Vitamin C is essential for preventing disease and ensuring bones, teeth, skin, and tendons are healthy. ■ It also helps with wound healing and preventing damage to cells.	Most fruits and vegetables, and potatoes. Best sources include oranges, blackcurrants, strawberries, spring greens, and green and red peppers.
Folate (a B vitamin, also known as folic acid)	■ This B vitamin ensures production of red blood cells. Folate helps to optimize cell growth and maintain the nervous system. ■ A lack of folate can result in folate-deficiency anaemia. ■ Folate cannot be stored within the body, so it must be present in the diet each day.	Most fortified breakfast cereals, dark green leafy vegetables (such as spinach), liver and kidney, oranges, yeast extract, wholemeal bread, and peanuts.
Iron	■ An essential mineral present in all body cells. ■ Plays a key role in enabling the transport of oxygen around the body via the red blood cells; helps to regulate cell growth. ■ Can be stored in the body, but a long-term lack results in iron-deficiency anaemia.	Red meat, liver, and kidney, oil-rich fish, such as sardines, eggs, dark green vegetables, wholegrains, such as brown rice, fortified breakfast cereals, peas, beans, lentils, and dried fruit.
Zinc	■ A key nutrient that helps the immune system to fight off invading pathogens, such as bacteria and viruses.	Lean meat, liver, kidney, canned oily fish, wholegrain cereals, nuts, eggs, milk, peas, and lentils.
Dietary fibre	■ Aids bowel efficiency by speeding up waste removal from the gut.	Wholegrain cereals and breads, pulses, vegetables, fresh and dried fruit, and seeds.

- Slower recovery time following operations or surgery.
- Skin problems, ulcers, and pressure sores (p.102).
- Muscle weakness, which increases the likelihood of falls.
- Difficulties moving and carrying out basic tasks of daily living.
- Tiredness, confusion, and irritability.

Drinking well

Recognizing thirst becomes more difficult as a person gets older, and therefore it is essential that drinks are regularly provided and encouraged throughout the day. Dehydration (p.53) is a common cause of admission to hospital among older people, as it can contribute to bladder infections, constipation, and bowel disorders, as well as to falls and confusion. It can also greatly increase the side effects of medication.

As a general rule, aim to offer between seven and eight glasses a day, but don't restrict this to just water. Drinks can also take the form of tea, fruit teas, coffee, milk, milkshakes, smoothies, or fresh fruit juices. By varying the drinks that you offer the person, you will help to enhance their appeal. Milk-based drinks can be useful, as they offer both fluid and

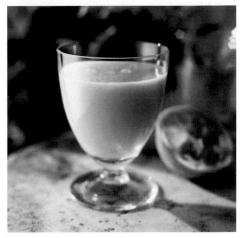

Nutritional boost
A glass of brightly coloured fruit juice looks instantly appealing and provides a boost of vitamins as well as essential fluid.

nutrients. It is particularly important to offer lots of fluid if the person you are looking after is constipated (p.51). If she is having problems swallowing (p.54), then fluid can be offered as thick nutritious soups or vegetable purées, ice lollies, sorbets, ice creams, jellies, or other watery foods. Ensure that appropriate cups and straws are available if drinking is becoming at all problematic for her (p.55).

VITAMIN D

Vitamin D is vital for bone health and is primarily processed by the body via the action of summer sunlight on the skin. Only a small amount is provided through foods.

- Good dietary sources include oil-rich fish, such as salmon, liver, egg yolk, and some fortified foods, but a person is unlikely to get enough vitamin D from diet alone.

- Anyone who is housebound, particularly if they are over 65, or who rarely goes outside should take a daily 10 microgram (mcg) supplement. Those with darker skins, who wear covering clothing, or who always wear sunscreen may also need a supplement.

- Supplements can be taken as a tablet or in the form of fish oils, such as cod liver oil.

- It is possible for a person to have too much vitamin D, and it is therefore important that only one form of the supplement should be taken at any one time and the recommended dosage is not exceeded.

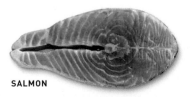

SALMON

MONITORING WEIGHT

It is important to be aware of fluctuations in a person's weight, as a discernible shift in either direction can bring with it various health risks. Among older people, being underweight is likely to contribute to more significant health problems than being overweight, as it is difficult to get enough nutrients if too little food is consumed. However, being overweight and eating too much food does not mean that someone automatically gets a good nutritional balance, as it is possible to be overweight and still be malnourished.

Spotting underweight

It can be difficult to spot weight loss if the person has been losing weight over a long period of time, and older people can often become very thin before this is treated as a significant risk to their health. You should be alert to any of the following warning signs of unintentional weight loss:

- Clothes become baggier.
- Bones are more visible under the skin.
- Belts are needed for trousers.
- Jacket shoulders no longer fit well.
- Rings and dentures fit more loosely.

The most accurate way of telling if the person is losing weight is to regularly measure her weight and height, enabling changes to be monitored over time and to identify whether she is underweight. For an average man, weight should not fall below 57kg (126lb); for women, it should not fall below 50kg (110lb). However, these indicators merely act as a guide. If the

BMI (BODY MASS INDEX)

The range of what constitutes a healthy BMI differs depending on a person's age; for those over 75 the range is much higher due to the increased risk of becoming underweight. The person's BMI can be plotted on the graph below by finding the point where her weight on the vertical axis intersects with her height on the horizontal axis. Ideally her BMI should fall within the healthy category for her age, as indicated on the graph by the coloured bands.

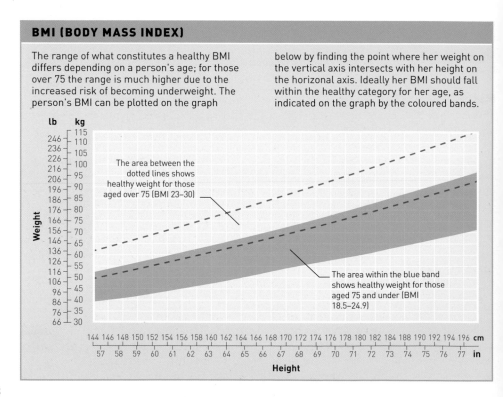

person is tall or of a naturally bigger build, then she could exceed the guide weight and still be underweight. Check any concern about weight loss with a doctor.

Weight loss can also be measured via changes in the person's BMI (body mass index), which is based on the relationship between weight and height. BMI is calculated by dividing the person's weight in kilograms (or pounds) with her height in metres (or inches) squared. The resulting BMI will indicate whether she is underweight, healthy, overweight, or obese. The criteria for those over 75 years old is different, and a higher range of BMI constitutes a healthy weight (opposite).

Older people will gradually lose height as they age. Therefore, for the BMI calculation, it is better to use their typical height when they were younger, if this is known. It may also be hard to measure the height of an older person if she has difficulty standing. In this situation, speak to a medical expert, who may be able to calculate the person's height from other body measurements.

Managing underweight

There can be a number of reasons why someone is losing weight, and it is first important to rule out a serious underlying disease, which might need medical investigation and possibly treatment. If an older person is underweight because she is simply not eating enough each day, there are some techniques you can use to help stimulate her appetite (see panel, right).

Spotting overweight

More than half of all adults in many western countries are overweight or obese. This means that they are heavier for their height than is considered good for their health. Adults of 75 and under are considered to be overweight if they have a BMI of 25 or more and obese if it is 30 or more. When people

STIMULATING THE APPETITE

Maintaining a person's appetite is important, especially if she is at risk of becoming underweight. There are various simple ways to help boost her appetite:

- She will feel hungrier if she is more active, and small amounts of exercise can be helpful, even if this is chair-based (p.96).

- Small, frequent meals and nutritious drinks can be useful in encouraging her to take in more calories across the day

- Ensure she is not consuming too many soft or sweetened drinks – these will be filling but provide few useful nutrients.

- Offer foods that look attractive, as most people tend to "eat with their eyes".

- Try serving her favourite foods, or foods from specific locations and cultures that remind her of happy past occasions.

- Strongly flavoured foods, such as those with added spices, or strongly flavoured cheeses, are known to boost the appetite.

- If alcohol is permitted, a small glass of sherry, wine, or beer before a meal is an appetite stimulant. Ensure that you check that alcohol is not contraindicated by any medication she may be taking.

- Instigating "cues" that a meal is coming can help to prepare older people who have dementia for a meal. Cues can be through stimulating the senses: sight, by getting tables ready; smell, by actively wafting cooking smells into the room; sound, by clattering pans; or touch, by involving the person in the meal's preparation.

get older, however, being thin is associated with the greatest risk to health, and it is generally agreed that a BMI of around 23 to 30 may be more appropriate for people over the age of 75. This provides a safety margin for any illness that may take hold where weight can drop quickly and significantly. This would mean that a woman aged 75 or under whose height measures 1.58m (62.4in) and who weighs 70kg (154lb), would be overweight, whereas a woman aged over 75 with, the same measurements would be considered to be a healthy weight.

» MONITORING WEIGHT

Risks to health of being overweight

People who are overweight or obese are at increased risk of high blood pressure, heart disease, type 2 diabetes, cancer, joint problems and arthritis, and breathing problems. They will also be more limited in their day-to-day activities, as they are likely to have decreased mobility and an increased need for care. A person who is overweight or obese and in need of care is going to be harder to lift, support, and bathe, and the person looking after them must be careful that her own health doesn't suffer as a result of this additional burden. Obesity is often linked with a poor diet, meaning that the person could be obese while also being undernourished. If obesity is having a significant negative impact on the daily quality of life, then specialist help should be sought.

Managing overweight

There are several ways to encourage a person to manage excessive weight or obesity (see panel, below). It is important

OVEREATING IN PEOPLE WITH DEMENTIA

Although weight loss is a common problem in people with dementia, overeating at certain stages of the disease may also occur.

- The person may have forgotten she has already eaten, and so eat twice.
- She may eat for comfort.
- She may suffer anxiety about future food supplies.
- She may be experiencing cravings for sweet foods, which can take hold at stages of dementia; the nutritional balance of meals can therefore become skewed.

It is important to consider how best to manage mealtimes in order to minimize these problems. Seek medical advice if necessary, especially if the person's health is suffering.

that the focus should always be on promoting a healthy lifestyle: encouraging the person to eat well to ensure she gets all the requisite nutrients, to be as active as possible, and to try to boost her mental wellbeing and social activity.

TIPS FOR MANAGING OVERWEIGHT

People may gain weight for a number of reasons, so there is not one simple solution. If a person needs to manage her weight, the main aim is to ensure that she eats no more calories each day than she uses up, but at the same time ensuring that she eats enough to provide all the necessary nutrients. To do this effectively, the best tips are:

- Cut out foods and drinks that provide calories but no nutrients, particularly any type of soft or alcoholic drink, as well as sweets or confectionery.
- Cut down on foods that provide lots of energy but are not essential, such as fat-based spreads, salad dressings, oils or fats used in cooking or on vegetables, and cream or dairy ice cream with desserts.

- Increase her daily fruit and vegetable intake at meals and snacks.
- Increase her intake of starchy foods, such as potatoes, pasta, rice, and bread, but make sure these are not served with added fat or sugar. Choose wholemeal varieties where possible, as they will be more filling.
- Offer smaller portions at mealtimes and use smaller plates and bowls.
- If the person becomes impatient before or between meals, offer slices of fruit and vegetables or a vegetable juice.
- Keep her active, as this reduces the time in which she may snack and increases her energy expenditure. Activity is also vital for both her physical and mental health.

SPOTTING MALNUTRITION

Malnutrition can have a wide range of effects on a person's physical as well as mental health (p.46). It is therefore important to recognize when someone may be at risk of becoming malnourished so that appropriate support can be given.

Warning signs

There are a number of key factors that are known to be related to undernutrition, particularly in older people:

■ **Losing interest in food** Older people commonly lose interest in eating and this is often the start of a nutritional decline. It may be caused by various factors, some of which can be managed and improved:
■ The person may be depressed or anxious and can be treated with talking therapies or medication.
■ The person may be in the early stages of dementia and it is vital to talk to her doctor about how to support and manage this.
■ The person may be uncomfortable when eating as a result of mouth pain, mouth ulcers, tooth pain, swallowing problems, wind, constipation, loose bowels, or another digestive condition. Seek treatment if you think any of these is a problem.
■ Low iron levels or thyroid problems can reduce appetite; check with her doctor.
■ The person may have psychological issues around food that may be related to dementia or another mental health issue. Take seriously comments related to food or appetite and seek help if necessary.
■ Side effects from medication can cause drowsiness or impact on the appetite, so it is worth asking for a medication review.

Changes in eating habits
If the person loses her appetite on a long-term basis, it may lead to a nutritional decline; any concerns should be discussed with a doctor.

■ **Bowel problems** More than 40 per cent of adults in the UK regularly suffer from constipation, and this increases significantly with age. Constipation in older people should be taken seriously, as it can lead to hospitalization and is often the precursor to much more serious problems. One of the main causes of constipation is consuming too little fluid and dietary fibre. However, there are a number of other factors that put someone at risk of constipation, and it is important to be aware of what they are in order to alleviate the problem. Factors that may increase the risk of constipation include:
■ A loss of mobility.
■ Taking medicines, such as tranquillizers, strong painkillers, and some medicines given to manage convulsions, tremors, and shaking. If new medicines are prescribed, always check with the person's doctor about any potential side effects.
■ Having a thyroid disorder, which may lead to slower gut movement.
■ Anxiety, for example if the person is having a change in routine or support.
■ Over-use of laxatives in the past, which may mean that a person is less able to function without stimulation.

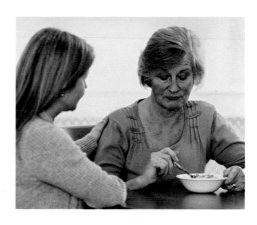

» SPOTTING MALNUTRITION

■ Poor dental health often results in a low-fibre diet as the person is likely to rely on soft-textured foods and avoid chewy, high-fibre foods, such as fruit and vegetables.

■ Often people think that if they eat less they will have fewer problems, but greater bulk is needed to reduce constipation.

■ **Change in mobility** If the person you are caring for suddenly loses her mobility, her food and drink intake and her overall health and wellbeing may be affected. Being less mobile means she will burn up less energy moving and so be less hungry, she may struggle to get food and drink when she wants it, or she might limit her choices to things that are easier to obtain or prepare. Reduced mobility means a person is at greater risk of constipation and also pressure sores (p.102), which require additional nutritional support to aid the healing process. Be alert to changes in a person's movement and ensure that she is encouraged to continue to eat well and be as active as she is able, for example through sitting exercises (p.96).

■ **Loss of independence in eating** Once someone starts to struggle with eating or loses the ability to feed herself completely, it can become very difficult to maintain motivation for eating well. This is one of the key factors associated with malnutrition in older people. There may be a number of reasons why someone struggles to eat independently:

■ Loss of ability to use cutlery, due to mental or physical impairment.

■ Tremor or shaking hands, making using cutlery more difficult.

■ Muscle weakness, loss of movement, or surgery on limbs.

■ Inability to sit up independently.

■ Confusion and wandering around during mealtimes.

It is important to consider how to ensure the person's independence is maintained as much as possible. This may be through offering her finger foods to avoid the need for cutlery (p.57), or it may be through using specialist equipment to make eating and drinking easier (p.55). The best option may be a combination of encouraging the person to eat independently while offering her support. The key is to help the person to maintain her autonomy in terms of what food she eats, how much she eats, and when she eats, so that she maintains some control and dignity at mealtimes.

■ **Plate waste** Regularly leaving food on the plate is one of the best indicators that a person may be at risk of entering a nutritional decline. If food portions that were typically eaten at a meal suddenly seem to be too big, snacks are declined, and there is an overall reduction in food eaten throughout the day, then the person may not be consuming enough energy and nutrients to meet her needs.

Making food more nutritious

If the person is eating a smaller volume of food than previously and she is either losing weight or is already underweight, it is important that the foods she does eat offer as much energy and nutrients as possible. There are simple and effective ways of adding nutritional value to meals and snacks and boosting energy:

■ Cream adds energy, fat, vitamins A, D, E, and B2 (riboflavin) to the diet. Cream can be stirred into porridge, soup, milky desserts, sauces, and hot drinks, as well as used in cakes or as a topping for puddings. Full-fat yoghurt and fromage frais can also be used, and soft high-fat cheeses, such as full-fat cream cheese or mascarpone, add an energy boost to dishes.

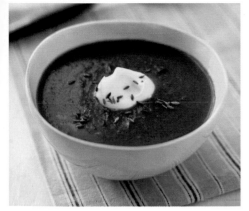

Extra calorific value
Fortifying foods can be a simple and effective way of meeting a person's nutritional needs. Adding a spoonful of thick cream to a nutritious soup gives an appetizing look as well as a calorific boost.

- Ordinary milk can be fortified by adding skimmed milk powder – this adds extra protein as well as other nutrients, such as calcium and phosphorus.
- Cheese and butter can be used in higher quantities and added to vegetables.
- Mayonnaise can be used in recipes, sandwiches, salads, vegetables, and dips.
- Chocolate nut spread and nut butters make good energy-dense toppings to spread onto toast or bread.
- Omelettes and scrambled eggs can have extra egg yolk added to provide more energy, protein, vitamins, and minerals.
- For vegans, or those with a dairy intolerance, purée tofu into calcium-fortified unsweetened soya milk.

The danger of dehydration

Dehydration occurs when a person's body loses more fluid than it takes in. As older people do not always recognize thirst efficiently, this can be a common problem. Dehydration can lead to urine infections and compacted faeces in the bowel, which can make incontinence worse (p.137) and have serious health consequences.

Certain circumstances can increase the likelihood of a person becoming dehydrated. These include habitually forgetting to drink, for example due to a condition such as dementia; struggling to access fluids independently and needing support in order to drink; having a tremor, which means a special cup or straw is needed; or requiring thickened drinks due to the risk of choking. Older people may also restrict their fluid intake over fears of incontinence, and it is important to encourage more fluid consumption when incontinence is an issue, as evidence shows that greater fluid intake is associated with better bladder control.

Promoting good drinking habits in the person you are looking after is vital, and there are various ways to encourage her fluid intake (p.47). Key to this is ensuring she drinks regularly throughout the day.

IMPORTANT!

Dehydration can range from mild to severe. It is crucial to be alert to any warning signs, as it may become a medical emergency if left untreated. In a case of mild to moderate dehydration, the person's condition can usually be rectified by increasing fluid intake. However, symptoms to look out for include:

- Dizziness and headaches.
- Fatigue.
- Dryness of the mouth, eyes, and lips.
- Infrequent urination.
- Dark, strong-smelling urine.

In a case of severe dehydration, the person requires immediate medical attention because, in extreme circumstances, dehydration can prevent efficient circulation of the blood. Symptoms to look out for include:

- Sagging skin.
- Sunken eyes.
- Blood in faeces or vomit.
- Rapid heartbeat.
- Seizures.

SWALLOWING AND EATING DIFFICULTIES

Eating difficulties may arise if someone has mouth problems or poor dental health; is recovering from surgery on the mouth, jaw, or neck; or has difficulty swallowing. Problems such as these must be carefully managed because, if the person's diet is suffering as a result, it can have a detrimental effect on overall health.

Swallowing difficulties

One of the key reasons that eating and drinking may become problematic is difficulty swallowing. This is a common problem after having a stroke; for people who have a degenerative illness, such as Parkinson's disease or multiple sclerosis (MS); for dementia sufferers; and in some forms of cancer that affect the head and neck. A speech and language therapist can assess swallowing capacity and suggest appropriate ways to manage the problem safely. People with swallowing difficulties are more likely to be undernourished or

dehydrated and are at risk of breathing in food particles to the lungs, which can lead to chest infections.

■ **Supporting someone with swallowing problems** The most common solution to a person's swallowing problem is to have the texture of her food and drink altered (p.57). This means offering foods of a naturally softer texture or, if swallowing is very problematic, puréed foods. It may also be necessary to give slightly thickened drinks, as this will slow the passage of fluid down the throat and decrease the risk of it entering the lungs. Thickening agents can be added to normal drinks.

A speech and language therapist can assess what texture is appropriate for each person and will explain how to obtain thickening agents to use in drinks.

A person with a swallowing difficulty may still be able to remain independent in her eating. However, there may be situations when assistance is required. See p.56 for advice on helping someone to eat.

Mouth problems

There are a number of reasons why someone may have a sore mouth or difficulty in chewing, for example poor dental health, gum problems, or physical problems with the jaw. If the person is struggling to chew, then she is likely to have a restricted diet, so any problem should be resolved as quickly as possible.

For mouth ulcers or sore patches in the mouth, a regular antiseptic mouthwash may be beneficial. If a person has sore gums or signs of gum disease, such as red, swollen gums or bleeding after brushing, encourage a visit to the dental hygienist. Visiting a dentist regularly is essential to

---

SIGNS OF SWALLOWING DIFFICULTY

If you have any concern about a potential swallowing problem, it is vital to seek advice from a health professional. There are some common signs to watch out for that may indicate a person is having difficulty:

- Coughing and choking before, during, or after swallowing.
- Frequent throat clearing.
- A gurgly or hoarse voice.
- Recurrent chest infections.
- Difficulty controlling food or drink in the mouth.
- If the person reports having difficulty in chewing or swallowing, or has feelings of an obstruction in the throat.

ensure that the greatest number of teeth can be maintained. A person's chewing ability is directly related to the number of teeth she has. If she is unable to brush her own teeth, ask her dentist or hygienist for advice on how to safely clean the person's mouth and teeth for her.

Maintaining good oral health is vital, as tooth decay and erosion can happen at any age. Advice on protecting teeth – through regular brushing with fluoride toothpaste and avoiding sugary or acidic foods and drinks between meals – applies to older people as well as younger ones.

Equipment to make eating easier

When a person is struggling to manage her cutlery, to physically keep food on the plate, or to keep her tableware steady, specially adapted equipment can be used to ease the eating process (see panel, below). An occupational therapist can advise you on different options. If, for example, the person finds it hard to grip securely, perhaps due to stiffness or reduced muscle control, it may be possible for her to use cutlery with a widened handle or a cup with enlarged handles. Slip-resistant mats or heavier-weight plates and bowls can help with controlling tableware, and attachable

SPECIAL EATING EQUIPMENT

ADAPTED UTENSIL	HOW IT CAN HELP
Cups with big handles	■ Cups or mugs are available with bigger handles or double handles, which can help the person hold them securely. ■ They are also available in different weights and materials: a weighted cup can prevent spillage; and a transparent cup helps someone see how much liquid remains inside.
Cutlery	■ Cutlery can be obtained in different shapes and materials. There can also be variation in the shape, size, and the angle of the handle: short-handled cutlery is easier to manage, while a thicker handle helps with grip.
Plates with safeguards	■ Plates and bowls can be fitted with attachable safeguards so food cannot fall off. Such plates can also be angled to aid getting food easily onto the fork or spoon.
Non-slip mats and plates	■ Non-slip mats can secure bowls and plates; dishes with non-slip bottoms are also available.
Insulated bowls	■ Bowls that keep food warm can help keep food at the right temperature for slow eaters.
One-way straws	■ One-way straws can help those with a weak suck or those who have difficulty in holding a cup.

» SWALLOWING AND EATING DIFFICULTIES

safeguards can be secured to plates and bowls to make it easier to manage the food. It is important to explore all these possibilities, as small adaptations can mean the person remains independent during mealtimes.

Helping someone to eat

It is a privilege to help someone eat, and a task that should be carried out with care and sensitivity. Remember that the person you are supporting is an adult and that you are helping her to eat and not passively "feeding" her. Encourage her to be as independent as possible and only help with those tasks that she is actively struggling with. For some people this might be cutting up food; for others the help required may be more substantial. Bear in mind that this is a two-way process that requires good communication and plenty of time. The key points to remember when helping someone to eat are:

- Make sure that the person you are helping is sitting upright and is fully prepared for the meal.
- Sit at eye level or slightly below the person you are helping. Position yourself either immediately in front of her or slightly to one side, so that you can maintain eye contact and communicate throughout.
- Use verbal prompts to explain every stage of the process. If the person is deaf, try to use gentle touch to alert her that food is coming, for example by stroking her arm gently before you start.
- Make sure the person knows what the meal is that you are offering and present it to her in small spoonfuls, developing a feeding rhythm so she can take the food, swallow it, and breathe.

HELPING PEOPLE WITH DEMENTIA TO EAT WELL

People with dementia may have particular problems at mealtimes, such as becoming confused or agitated. If you are caring for someone with dementia, it is very important to understand how her condition affects her, so you can give appropriate support. Seek advice from her doctor or a medical specialist to better prepare yourself and to help her.

Older people with dementia are at great nutritional risk, and thinness is extremely common. This is primarily caused by not eating enough rather than the disease itself, and if someone is losing weight, follow all the tips on pp.52–53 to promote extra energy and nutrient intake. The key points when helping someone with dementia to eat well are:

- Maintain a quiet and calm atmosphere – it is essential to allow the person to focus on the process of eating.
- Provide cues that meals are coming, via the sights, sounds, and smells of cooking.
- Eat with the person so that you can model eating and offer encouragement.
- Be aware of any difficulty using cutlery and adapt her diet or equipment as necessary.

- Encourage the person to retain control of the meal by indicating what she wants to eat next and when. This may be vocally or just through a gentle tap on your arm.
- Stay focused on the task – if there are others in the room, don't talk to them over the person's head, and keep the process as calm and quiet as possible.
- Think about the equipment you use when helping someone to eat. If you find the person is struggling with certain aspects of the meal, consider what specialist equipment (p.55) might be best employed to help her, or seek advice from an occupational therapist or the doctor.

SPECIAL DIETARY NEEDS

There are a number of different special dietary needs that may determine the type and amount of food that a person is able to eat, or even the texture of food that can be eaten safely. Dietary needs can range from being diabetic to being able only to cope with puréed foods. Once the types of food that are eaten start to be restricted, it becomes harder to take in the daily requirement of energy and nutrients. Extra care should therefore be taken to ensure sufficient nutritional content is maintained.

Altered-texture diets

Changing the texture of the person's diet becomes necessary if she is unable to chew properly or manipulate food in her mouth (p.54). Depending on the level of difficulty, the person may require either soft-textured or puréed foods. Specialist advice should be sought before making any significant dietary changes.

■ **Soft-textured foods** These are foods that can be mashed easily with a fork, or that are easy to break up with the tongue and require little chewing, such as scrambled

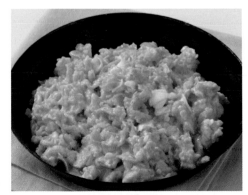

Soft-textured food
People who can no longer chew effectively may need to eat soft-textured foods, such as scrambled eggs, which require minimal chewing.

eggs. Many meals can be adapted to be soft-textured by simply mashing or finely chopping the foods, cooking foods until they are softer, and adding sauces so that food can move more smoothly down the throat. Crumbly foods should be avoided.

■ **Puréed foods** These should be totally smooth and require no chewing, so the food forms into a soft mass in the mouth that can be easily swallowed. Once a person needs puréed food, it is very difficult to provide enough energy each day, and at least five small meals are likely to be needed. Purées must be fortified with additional energy or protein so they are nutrient rich. Typical additions include full-fat dairy products, skimmed milk powder, or calorific sweeteners, such as honey or jam. Liquidizing the purée with fluid should be avoided, as this will merely dilute its nutritional content.

Finger foods

If a person develops a condition that affects her ability to hold, manipulate, or even recognize cutlery, she may well benefit from a finger food diet. The aim is to remove the need for cutlery in order to prolong independent eating. Finger foods need to be easy to hold, well-structured, of a suitable temperature, and served in bite-sized chunks. Examples include quiches, sandwiches, and kebabs. It is vital that a good variety of finger foods from different food groups are consumed to ensure the person maintains a balanced diet.

Diabetic diets

Diabetes is caused by an inability to regulate blood sugar levels and may need to be treated with injections of the hormone insulin, by medicines that control rises in blood sugar, or through changes in

» SPECIAL DIETARY NEEDS

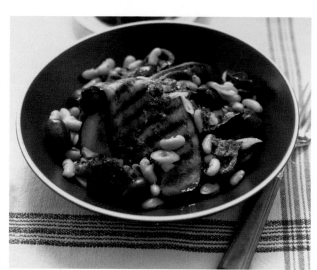

Adding protein
Beans provide an excellent source of protein for vegetarians and vegans, and can easily be added to many dishes or used as the basis for a meal.

Vegetarian and vegan diets

It is easy to get all necessary nutrients from a varied vegetarian diet that includes dairy products and eggs. However, vegans must include a source of vitamin B12 in their diet, as this nutrient will not be provided when no animal products are eaten. Vitamin B12 can be obtained from fortified soya milks, textured vegetable proteins, and yeast extracts. Iodine and vitamin B2 (riboflavin) are also lower in vegan diets, and, while these nutrients can be found in non-animal products, many vegans take a daily supplement to ensure adequate amounts.

the diet and increased exercise. Most diabetics eat a normal healthy diet without needing to buy specialist foods. Reducing sugars and fat intake is recommended, and eating regularly across the day is important if someone is on insulin. A health professional will give advice on how to manage meals and snacks alongside insulin and other medicines. Key points of dietary advice for diabetics include:

- Sweets, soft drinks, cakes, and biscuits should be avoided; if small amounts are consumed, these should be eaten with meals, not as snacks.
- Diabetes carries a risk of heart disease, so a diet full of fruits, vegetables, oil-rich fish, lean meat, reduced-fat dairy products, and wholegrain cereals is recommended.
- Diabetics are better able to manage their condition if they are active, so encourage as much activity as the person is able to do.
- Always check labels for any added sugar content in flavoured waters, mixer drinks, fruit juice and fruit juice drinks, energy drinks, and snacks and ready meals.

FOOD SENSITIVITY

Food sensitivity can refer to either an allergy or an intolerance that a person may have to a particular food or food component.

- With an allergy, any amount of the trigger food causes a rapid and potentially violent reaction, and may require an emergency response from a carer (p.187).

- Intolerances to foods or components of foods – such as lactose, which is the sugar in dairy products, or gluten, the protein in wheat, barley, rye, and oats – mean these foods must be avoided, to prevent digestive discomfort through bloating or cramps. Lactose- and gluten-free foods are widely available but can be expensive, Instead, try to plan meals with foods that are acceptable.

WHEN FOOD IS NOT ENOUGH

Sometimes it is not possible to sustain a person's nutritional needs through diet alone. This may be due to an ongoing condition or dietary restrictions, or something acute (short-term), such as an inability to eat following surgery, an illness or infection, or an accident. If the person is at risk of not eating enough, she may require nutritional supplements.

Vitamin and mineral supplements

Sometimes additional amounts of a vitamin or mineral are needed, for example if the person has an iron deficiency. Always check with the person's doctor before you give supplements, as too much of most nutrients may be as harmful as too little.

Food supplements

These are usually milkshake-type drinks that provide energy (calories), protein, fat, and other essential nutrients. A typical food supplement carton provides about 15 per cent of an older person's daily energy and nutrient needs, so it is vital that they are used as supplements to other foods and drinks, not as a substitute for a day's food.

Food supplements are designed for short-term use and people often tire of them quickly, so it is important to encourage a return to a normal diet as soon as possible. Supplements are easily contaminated if left lying around for long periods, as they have a high nutrient content, making them attractive to bacteria. Always follow the manufacturer's storage instructions carefully and discard any food supplement after its use-by date.

Artificial feeding

If the ability to eat or swallow becomes very problematic, a decision may be made to provide the person with food via a tube. This may be inserted through the nose (a nasogastric tube), into the stomach (a PEG tube), or, if the person is extremely ill, directly into the bloodstream (parenteral nutrition). Artificial feeding may be a short-term solution after illness or surgery and is initially begun in hospital. You'll be given advice for ongoing care in the home and offered community support by a health professional. The tube feeds are provided by the hospital, and instructions on storage and usage must be carefully followed to avoid risk of contamination.

If the person is eventually able to return to a normal diet, a health professional will offer advice on how to gradually reintroduce her to solid foods.

NUTRITIONAL SUPPLEMENT OPTIONS

SUPPLEMENT TYPE	DIETARY NEED
Vitamin and mineral supplements	Likely to be offered when a person has a specific nutritional lack, such as iron deficiency. They are to be taken as prescribed by a doctor.
Food supplements	May be prescribed if there is concern over someone's energy and nutrient intake, and a supplement is needed for a short period.
Non-oral method of feeding	In extreme circumstances, if a person cannot eat, all nutritional needs are provided via a tube into the nose, stomach, or bloodstream.

THE IMPORTANCE OF MEALTIMES

Eating is an integral part of everyone's life. As well as providing sustenance, eating gives structure to the day and it is a natural outlet for humans as social beings, offering a source of pleasure, memory, and comfort. Mealtimes are particularly important for those who are housebound or have limited moblility, as they become key focal points for each day.

Most people eat full meals at breakfast, lunch, and dinner and frequently snack in between, but if a person is elderly or ill, then the arrangement of meals and snacks is likely to vary, depending on the person's requirements and lifestyle.

Eating well across the day

How someone chooses to eat across the day will vary, and it is important to ensure that meals are offered at times the person is used to and wants to eat. Some people want a main meal in the middle of the day, while others prefer it in the evening. Some prefer smaller meals but more snacks across the day. Whatever the pattern of eating, ensure that good food and drink choices are always available and don't stick to rigid routines if these are not helping the person to eat well.

■ **Breakfast** For some people breakfast may be when they are most alert and hungry, so this can be a good time to offer the biggest meal. Typical breakfast foods of bread and wholegrain cereals are high in fibre and B vitamins, and eggs can provide a range of useful nutrients in a small volume of food. Porridge with fruit is a good, simple breakfast, and fresh fruit or fruit juice served with cereals may aid iron absorption. There is, however, no reason why breakfast-style foods have to be eaten, so follow the lead of the person you support on what she would like to eat at this time.

Vitamin boost
Fruits are excellent snacks that provide a nutritional boost as well as vital fluids.

■ **Main meals** The largest meals typically provide the most nutrients each day. If these are missed, it can be difficult to catch up on their nutritional content at other times. Main meals should be varied, offer a good source of protein, such as meat (or meat substitute), fish, nuts, soya, or egg; a source of carbohydrate, such as potato, pasta, or rice; and one or two different vegetables. Desserts made with fruit and milk can add important nutrients.

■ **Snacks** The best snacks provide useful nutrients rather than empty calories. Good examples include yoghurts, fresh fruit, crackers spread with pâté, dips, dried fruit, smoothies, and cakes or buns that contain fruit or vegetables, such as carrot cake.

■ **Drinks** Make sure drinks are regularly offered. If someone eats well, soft drinks will not compromise her nutrient intake, but if there are concerns about her nutrition, it is better to offer more nutritious drinks based on milk or fresh fruit juice.

Who can help?

Older people living in their own homes may be offered support from care assistants (p.22). Care assistants offer a variety of support, but most will have had little training in supporting someone to eat well.

It may be helpful to talk to the care assistant about how to provide the best nutritional care for the person you are looking after. This could be advice on the sort of food to buy or prepare, how to encourage eating or drinking, how to monitor any poor eating habits in the person, and, crucially, when to alert others if there is a suspected problem with levels of nutrition.

■ **Community meals** If the person becomes unable to make a main meal each day, she may be offered a community meal from the "meals on wheels" service. This may be free or subsidised, and can be delivered either hot and ready to eat or frozen and ready for the person to heat up herself. Community meals are likely to be a better choice than other frozen ready meals, and a hot meal delivery every day provides a focal point as well as social interaction. It is important to maintain a good dialogue between any carers to ensure community meals are received and eaten safely. Keep a watchful eye on the person's nutritional status even if she does have community meals, as these alone may not provide adequate nutrition if she is becoming undernourished.

■ **Lunch clubs and other group settings** Eating with others often stimulates people to eat better, and many enjoy attending a daily or weekly lunch club. These are often situated in churches or community centres and run by volunteers. Your local council can provide a list of all the lunch clubs in the area. Many provide transport and are a lifeline to isolated older people. In many areas, there are also specialist lunch clubs for people with dementia and for those with specific cultural backgrounds.

■ **Home deliveries** A person may choose to have shopping delivered to her home and can be helped to do this via community shopping services or the internet, if she has access to this or can be assisted.

Communal meals
Eating meals with others offers social stimulus to someone who is usually alone at mealtimes, be it with a family group or an organized club.

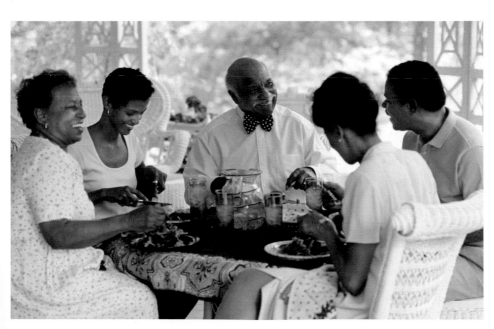

PUTTING EATING WELL INTO PRACTICE

There are a number of things you can do to enhance the person's enjoyment of her meals and to ensure that as much as possible of the food offered is eaten. Just because a person has a reduced appetite or requires help with eating does not mean that her criteria for good food is lessened.

Considerable research into the eating environment for people with dementia has been conducted, and shows that recreating a familiar dining setting – one that the person has been used to in previous years – encourages better eating. This may mean using a tablecloth, providing salt and pepper pots or napkins that the person remembers, using familiar crockery, and even including items on the table that are not in use but that stimulate memories of the past, such as teapots and tea cosies.

Maximizing enjoyment at mealtimes

It is important to make sure the person is ready for a meal, as small issues, such as needing the toilet, or not having glasses or a hearing aid in place, can spoil the dining experience. Try to consider any relevant criteria before you begin:

■ If a person's eyesight is poor, choose tableware that stands out – a coloured plate or a plate with a coloured edge can help it to be more easily identified.

■ For some people, eating requires concentration, so avoid any distractions, such as a loud television or radio.

■ People who struggle with eating may find that having someone eat with them can help to keep them motivated.

■ Communal eating (p.61) can stimulate the appetite; if a group of people are going to be eating together, a round table can encourage interaction.

LOOKING AFTER YOURSELF

Being a carer can be very demanding and can result in ignoring your own own health and wellbeing. In order to be able to offer good care, you need to be fit and well yourself:

■ Eat well every day – you can't make up for a few days' poor eating with one good day or one good meal.

■ Exercise as much as you can – every little bit helps, and walking is the easiest and best exercise for everyone.

■ Try to maintain a normal body weight and seek help if you become overweight.

■ Seek help and support if things are getting on top of you, especially if you think your own nutritional health is suffering.

■ Avoid unnecessary snacking. Many carers find they gain weight, as they become more sedentary and snack more as they try to encourage someone else to eat. Being careful not to snack unnecessarily or unhealthily, and building activity into your day, can help guard against weight gain.

■ Consider any outdoor space and how accessible it is. Alfresco dining in good weather can be a refreshing change.

■ Special occasions are often tightly linked with eating, and offering food associated with festive or religious occasions can help to encourage a person to eat.

Food presentation

Presentation of food and drink can often encourage – or discourage – eating. Making food look attractive on the plate, not overwhelming the person with huge portions, and thinking about what foods complement each other can all boost the appetite. Inventive touches, such as serving drinks as "cocktails" or ice creams in cones, can encourage reluctant eaters.

FOOD HYGIENE AND FOOD SAFETY

Older people and those who are ill are at greater risk of food poisoning. It is therefore essential to adhere to basic food safety guidance when preparing meals.

Storing food

Correct storage of food and an awareness of the length of time different foods can be kept is vital. Harmful bacteria can transfer from raw foods to cooked foods if they are not stored apart, and this is one of the main causes of food poisoning. Following basic storage guidelines will help to keep food fresh for longer, maximizing its usage:

■ Food that can go off at room temperature should not be left out for more than two hours. Refrigerate it at a temperature below 5°C (41°F).

■ Cool and refrigerate leftovers within two hours; eat within 48 hours.

■ Eggs should be kept in the fridge.

■ Food stocks should be rotated so that the oldest is used first. Any food past its use-by date should be thrown away.

■ Only buy pasteurized dairy products.

Preparing food

Maintaining basic rules of hygiene helps prevent the spread of harmful bacteria:

■ Always wash your hands and ensure utensils and surfaces are clean.

■ Wash all fruit and vegetables thoroughly.

■ Heat food until it is piping hot or around 70°C (158°F) for at least two minutes, and then allow it to cool before serving.

■ Avoid serving raw or rare meats and fish.

Eating safely

If the person you are looking after suffers from any swallowing difficulties or may be at risk of choking, never leave her alone while eating, and ensure that any carer in charge of her knows what to do in the event of her choking (p.178). If the person is in a wheelchair, always check that the wheels are locked when she is eating, so it cannot move if accidentally knocked. If the person suffers from any food allergies, ensure that anyone who supports her is aware of this and knows how to manage any reaction that may occur (p.187).

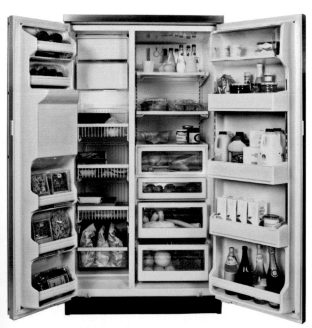

Storing food in the fridge

A neatly stocked fridge is easy to manage and reduces the chance of products festering in the back and spreading bacteria to other foods.

4

SOCIAL AND
MENTAL WELLBEING

■ GETTING OUT OF THE HOUSE ■ LEISURE ACTIVITIES
■ COMMUNICATION ■ STAYING MENTALLY ALERT
■ COPING AFTER A STROKE

GETTING OUT OF THE HOUSE

Encouraging and helping the person you are caring for to remain active and socially engaged can be challenging, but has many benefits. It helps him to maintain his fitness and ability to carry out daily activities, and provides important social contact, relaxation, and a sense of enjoyment and fulfilment. Getting out of the house together is beneficial for you both, too, as it provides a refreshing change of scene if you spend a lot of time indoors.

You will need to prepare for any outing you take together. Think in advance about the route, and factors such as whether there are hills, places to stop and rest, and toilet facilities. It is worth taking any medication the person needs with you in case you are delayed, as well as layers of clothing and a drink and snack.

Getting out locally

Encourage the person to take short trips out with you whenever possible. Simply walking up the road to get a paper or do a small grocery shop will help to keep him healthy and aware of his environment, and it helps to prevent social isolation.

Bear in mind that even short trips, such as a walk around the block or to the local park, require a degree of planning and an assessment of any risks. Keep your phone with you in case of an emergency. Think, too, about whether you will need to cross busy roads and if there are places to sit for a rest.

If you are pushing a wheelchair, are you confident you can manoeuvre it up and down kerbs (p.93)? Try to avoid high pavements without dropped kerbs. If you feel there are too many difficult-to-negotiate kerbs, contact your council to see if these can be altered. Take along a rain cover for the wheelchair if the weather is changeable. If the person you are caring for has an electric wheelchair or scooter, he is probably fairly competent using it outside, but he may still need reassurance and will probably appreciate an extra pair of eyes to watch for traffic.

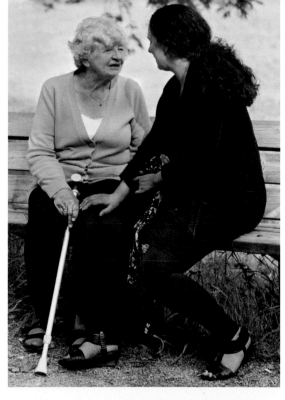

A change of scene
Getting out daily, to the local park or nearby shops, is worth the effort, providing stimulation, gentle exercise, and a welcome mental boost.

If you're planning a trip to the local shopping centre, check whether the centre offers a day rental of wheelchairs and scooters if needed. Most supermarkets now provide wheelchair-accessible trolleys that are pushed in front of a wheelchair, enabling the person to continue taking an active role in his shopping.

Using the car

If you are using the car for a longer journey or an outing and the person you are caring for has reduced mobility, ensure that the passenger seat is pushed back to give him plenty of room to manoeuvre and that the back of the seat is fairly upright. An extra cushion can provide comfort, and simple devices such as a swivel cushion (p.88) make getting in and out of the car easier for wheelchair users. Another useful gadget is a portable handle that enables people with restricted mobility to get into and out of a car independently.

Don't park too close to a pavement on the passenger side, as the raised surface makes it harder for the passenger to get out and stand up. Ideally, find a flat area, or stop away from the pavement so he can get out more easily, then re-park your car.

In the UK, "blue badges" for disabled parking areas can be applied for on behalf of your passenger. Usually, the person needs to be assessed first by an occupational therapist or doctor to acquire a badge.

Using public transport

If you are planning to use public transport, work out your journey in advance to reduce potential stress. Make sure you have up-to-date timetables for buses and trains, avoid travelling during busy times, and build in time to stop and rest when planning which

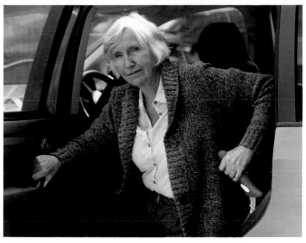

Handy aid
A portable handle that fits securely into the frame of a car makes it easier to get in or out of the car. It can be used on either side of the car.

bus or train to catch. Check, too, whether an elderly or disabled person is entitled to a discount card. You may also need to ask in advance about wheelchair access and to request help if necessary.

Some areas of the UK offer a community "dial-a-bus" service to the nearest shopping centre, providing a door-to-door service, usually with wheelchair lift access.

MEETING OTHERS

Getting involved in local events and activities can have significant benefits for an elderly person or someone with limited mobility. Group activities provide good opportunities for socializing, in turn reducing isolation and boosting confidence and self-esteem.

- Check out local day centres and lunch clubs, which often organize day outings.
- Tea dances are held in many areas and offer a great opportunity to socialize.
- Exercise and swimming groups for elderly people help to maintain mobility and fitness.
- Bridge clubs, art classes, and hobby-based groups provide stimulation and company.

LEISURE ACTIVITIES

Many hobbies and activities can still be enjoyed when a person becomes less able, although extra planning may be needed and the activity may need adapting.

Encourage the person to try a simple task first before moving on to a more complex one. This avoids a sense of failure, which could deter him from continuing with an activity. Be prepared to provide help to complete a task or to assist with more difficult areas.

Indoor hobbies and activities

Keeping up with hobbies and favourite activities can be challenging if a person has poor eyesight or reduced manual dexterity that affects his capacity to read and write or to manipulate objects. Fortunately, there are many aids available that can help (see panel, opposite).

■ **Jigsaws** Doing jigsaws helps to maintain hand function and also uses mental skills. Large-print jigsaws with as few as 40 pieces are available.

■ **Painting and drawing** If a person enjoys painting and drawing, he may enjoy adult colouring books, which are similar to painting by number but have larger areas for colouring in and can be used with paints, crayons, or chalks.

■ **Puzzles** Large-print versions of crosswords, wordsearches, and sudoku are widely available, and are ideal for maintaining mental and visual skills. There are easier versions for those with mental impairments.

■ **Craft kits** These can be satisfying and stimulating. Look for kits such as wooden nest boxes and doorknob hangers that are assembled, then decorated, and make useful presents. Egg cups and plant boxes can be painted, and numerous other "painting" kits are available. Try to find crafts that have some meaning and relevance to the person.

■ **Knitting and sewing** These pastimes can provide meaningful activity for people with limited mobility. If the person has poor manual dexterity, use simple patterns and lightweight wools when knitting. Smaller projects may be easier to manage. Easy-to-handle larger pins are useful, and there are knitting aids for one-handed use. If knitting proves to be too difficult or causes pain in the arms and hands, it is possible to pad out a crochet hook to aid grip and reduce pressure on joints. Thicker tapestry needles rather than embroidery needles are easier to use, and a sewing stand can help. For people with poor vision, sewing can be continued or learned with the help of equipment such as a needle threader, as well as good task lighting and magnifiers.

Gardening

Gardens and gardening are a common source of enjoyment for many people, whether simply relaxing outside or maintaining the garden.

Various aids are available to help those who find gardening more of a challenge but wish to continue with the lighter tasks. Look for lightweight tools and raise flower beds or pots if possible. Check that garden benches and seats aren't too low, and ensure that paths are level.

Active leisure pursuits

More physical pursuits, such as dancing, walking, and swimming (for the more mobile), are a common source of enjoyment. It's worth helping the person you are caring for to keep up with these activities, using aids if necessary (p.79).

AIDS FOR LEISURE ACTIVITIES

EQUIPMENT	DESCRIPTION AND PURPOSE
Book rests and book holders	■ A book rest (right) is ideal for those with poor grip. ■ Book holders on a stand are available for wheelchair users. 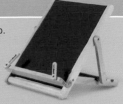
Magnifiers 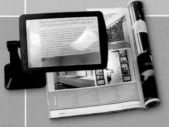	■ Many types of magnifier are available, including hands-free magnifying glasses that are supported against the body or that have a stand (left). ■ Some magnifiers have a built-in light source or feature high-digital magnification and run on batteries or plug in to a socket.
Easy-grip paintbrushes	■ Specialized paintbrushes with chubby grips and short handles are easier to manage for people who have a weak grip.
Writing aids 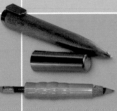	■ Large-grip pens (left) or chunky pencils are easier to hold for people with poor grip. ■ You can buy grips that fit over a pen or pencil, or you can wrap an elastic band or piece of foam tubing around a pen or pencil to create your own grip.
Knitting aids	■ Larger knitting needles (right) are easier to use for people with poor manual dexterity. ■ Craft tool holders that can be fixed to a table or chair arm and hold a knitting needle or other craft tool in place are useful for people who have the use of only one hand.
Needle threader  	■ An automatic needle threader makes threading a needle easier for people with poor vision.
Gardening aids	■ A lightweight garden kneeler/seat (right) can be positioned either way up and is useful for people who cannot stand for long. ■ Easy-grip handles that fix onto existing tools reduce the strain on the upper limbs. ■ Long-handled tools reduce the need to stretch or bend. 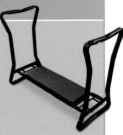

COMMUNICATION

It's important for the person you are caring for to maintain social contact with you and others. You may find that you need to adapt the way in which you communicate with him so that he can hear and understand you and you can understand him in turn. As the main carer, you will have inside knowledge and understanding of the person's communication skills and may need to be on hand to interpret for visitors and health professionals.

Adapting how you communicate

The person might have hearing or sight problems or a mental impairment, such as dementia, that means you need to tailor your communication, for example by relying on non-verbal cues (see panel). Someone who has had a stroke and suffered brain damage will have specific difficulties and needs (p.74). Re-evaluating your methods of communication may make you feel awkward and uneasy at first, but being able to understand each other is key to your relationship and the effectiveness of your care, so it's important that you adapt.

It is very frustrating for the person being cared for to feel misunderstood. As the

---

ENHANCING COMMUNICATION

Try the following to improve communication between you and the person you care for:

- Pay attention to body language and gestures.
- Use your tone of voice to emphasize meaning.
- Make eye contact when you speak, and don't stand over someone in a wheelchair or bed: come down to his level.
- Speak more slowly, and use shorter, simpler sentences.

---

carer, your reaction to his physical or mental difficulties may affect your communication, which in turn can affect how he responds.

Try to be aware of this and provide reassurance that you recognize his needs through touch, holding his hand, and gently encouraging him. Asking him which communication strategies work best can enhance his dignity and sense of inclusion.

Thinking about body language

When verbal communication is difficult, you need to pay even more attention to body language – how you both communicate with your eyes, facial expressions, gestures, touch, and posture. For you as a carer, making eye contact, smiling, touching, and adopting a relaxed, open posture are all reassuring. Be aware of the other person's body language, too. If he

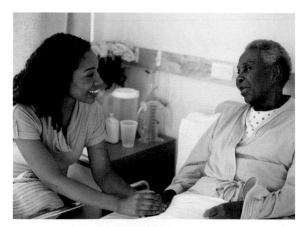

Good communication
Making eye contact, touching, and using positive body language are helpful in letting a person know that you empathize with her.

avoids eye contact, this could indicate low self-esteem and confidence. If he turns away from you, is he feeling angry or depressed? Watch out, too, for unusually laboured movements that could indicate he is in pain. Checking these non-verbal cues helps avoid misunderstandings.

Choosing a hearing aid

If the person you are caring for has impaired hearing, a hearing aid may help by making sounds clearer and louder. There is a range of hearing aids to choose from that are available in the UK on the NHS.

Most hearing aids are battery-operated, and normally are worn either behind the person's ear, in the outer ear, or in the actual ear canal.

You will be guided and advised by a trained specialist as to the most suitable hearing aid. While those inside the outer ear and ear canal are the most discreet, they are mainly suitable for those with mild to moderate hearing loss. Those worn outside the ear, which are larger, are most likely to be recommended for more severe

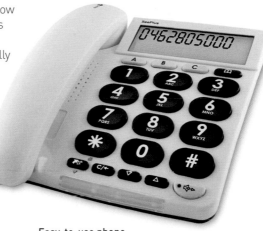

Easy-to-use phone
Clear displays, flashing ring alerts, and large, easy-to-press buttons help to make telephones more user-friendly for those with impaired hearing or vision.

hearing problems. Cochlear implants – small electronic devices surgically positioned under the skin – are available for those with more profound hearing loss.

Using the telephone

Most hearing aids have a setting that helps to filter out background noise while using the telephone. Known as a T coil, this acts like a wireless loudspeaker. Check, though, that the phone is compatible with the hearing aid; otherwise there will be "feedback", whereby amplified sound travels back into the hearing aid's microphone. Phones that are compatible with hearing aids have handy volume controls. It is also possible to purchase portable amplifiers that fit on existing handsets, or plug-in amplifiers to boost the volume of a standard phone.

Other useful features on phones include visual aids, for example flashing lights that alert the hard of hearing to an incoming call. For people with hearing and visual problems, there are phones with a vibrating pad alert that can be placed close by.

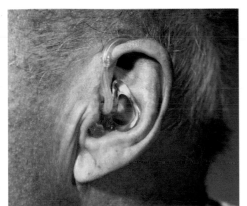

Using a hearing aid
A hearing aid enhances sounds, helping the wearer more easily take part in conversations and to feel connected to his surroundings.

STAYING MENTALLY ALERT

As people live longer, it has become increasingly important to keep body and mind healthy and active. Exercise, good diet, reduced alcohol intake, not smoking, and taking medication as prescribed help to keep us mentally and physically well. Socializing and enjoying company also help to ensure wellbeing. While gradual changes with age are natural – a reduction in hearing and vision, forgetting things, or being slower to learn new skills – intelligence does not diminish. If you are caring for an elderly person, bear in mind that he may simply need more time, flexibility, and motivation to achieve tasks.

Healthy body, healthy mind

There is an important link between physical and mental health. You can help an older person to stay mentally alert by encouraging him to do the following:

■ **Stay physically active** Encourage the person to stay as active as possible (pp.78–103). Being physically active strengthens bones and muscles, helps to lower blood pressure (reducing the likelihood of a stroke), increases energy levels, and reduces the risk of depression. More energy helps coordination, balance, and reaction times, and also increases

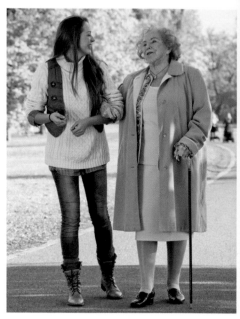

Exercise for the body and mind
As well as being a good way of staying mobile, a gentle daily walk sustains energy levels and provides a mental boost.

mental alertness, which in turn assists memory problems.

■ **Eat healthily** A balanced, nutritious diet helps to keep energy levels up and avoid listlessness and depression. Conversely,

---

HELPING SOMEONE TO STAY MENTALLY ACTIVE

Ensure the environment and lifestyle of the person you are caring for maximizes his mental health:

■ Help him to find ways to relax and reduce stress. Making time to unwind, perhaps while engaged in a hobby, can help to alleviate depression and anxiety.

■ Encourage him to maintain social contacts. Avoiding isolation is important for wellbeing. Maintaining religious connections if these have meaning can be beneficial as the

church or group may provide a supportive network, often carrying out home visits to housebound members of the congregation.

■ Keep him stimulated, to help mental alertness. A simple change in routine allows the brain to learn new patterns. This may be a minor change, such as trying a new recipe or going on a different outing. However, when caring for a person with dementia, take care when introducing a new task, as a change of routine can cause stress and upset.

overeating can cause, or contribute to, depression, reduce energy levels (both physical and mental), and increase the risk of high cholesterol and diabetes. Boost mental function by encouraging the person to eat "brain foods" such as fish oils, which contain essential minerals and vitamins, and to include plenty of fresh fruit and vegetables in the diet. Supplements may be helpful in some cases (p.59).

- **Avoid alcohol and smoking** Encourage the person to drink alcohol in moderation or not at all, and not to smoke. Check, too, whether alcohol or tobacco causes side effects with medications.
- **Maintain good dental hygiene** Looking after the teeth and gums is essential for good oral health; moreover, some studies indicate that there is a link between gum disease and some types of dementia.

Dementia and memory problems

Memory problems can be complex and vary from occasional forgetfulness to being unable to remember loved ones' names or even to recognize them. This can be hard for you as a carer and can make caring an exhausting and repetitive process.

As memory deteriorates, there are many techniques that can be used to try to help him maintain memory (see panel, right). However, it is often the case that memory continues to deteriorate and the person will no longer be able to function safely without you.

If the person's memory is very poor, memory books with photos and cuttings, or recording memories on a CD, can encourage conversation and inform visitors and younger family members. Continue to enjoy easy games like dominoes, and

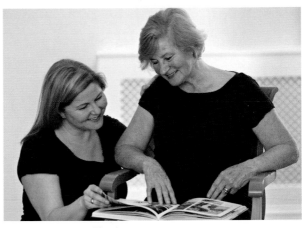

Familiar faces
Looking through treasured photo collections is a pleasurable experience and provides a useful reminder of friends and family.

encourage the person to listen to music and to dance. Simple activities, such as sitting in the kitchen while dinner is being prepared or stirring a bowl, can help the person feel part of a normal routine.

HELP FOR MEMORY PROBLEMS

After a stroke, or in the early stages of dementia, there are several things you can do to help a person deal with memory problems:

- Help him keep to a routine.
- Keep keys, money, and the phone in designated places; if necessary, label items.
- Leave a pad by the phone for the person to write down information.
- Encourage the person to carry a notebook with reminders or shopping lists in it.
- Use large calendars or wipe-down boards to leave messages.
- Play word games, such as scrabble and wordsearches, and cards and puzzles to exercise memory.
- Encourage the person to repeat words if he has trouble remembering. Alternatively, try asking him to visualize an item if he is struggling to find a word, as visual memory is more efficient.

COPING AFTER A STROKE

When difficulties with a relative, partner, or friend come on suddenly, as is the case with a stroke, you can feel unprepared, shocked, and unsure of how to help. You will need to learn how best to communicate with the person. There are also many activities that you as the carer can encourage and help him to do to resume his independence as far as possible.

Communication after a stroke

You may be unsure how to re-establish your previous speaking relationship with someone who has had a stroke and suffered brain damage. There may be complex mental and physical impairments, for example the person may find it difficult to form clear words and may not understand what you are saying as his mental processing has been affected by the stroke. These problems can be short- or long-term.

A person who has particular problems with speech and/or understanding, as well as with swallowing and writing, may be offered an assessment and services from a speech and language therapist. This will be arranged through the hospital or the person's own doctor. Once the type of brain damage has been identified, the therapist can work to improve the person's communication skills.

You will need to pay attention to how you communicate with the person, and make adaptations where necessary (see panel, above). Be especially sensitive if you need to discuss issues with a health professional about the person you are caring for that you don't want him to hear. Move to another room; even if he is unable to communicate verbally in a clear way, he may be able to understand the general meaning of what you are saying.

TIPS FOR COMMUNICATING

If you are caring for someone who has had a stroke and suffered brain damage, try the following to improve communication:

- Face the person and speak slowly and clearly; summarize and repeat the main points to check he understands.

- Turn off televisions and radios to reduce the amount of distracting background noise.

- Listen carefully and give the person more time to articulate his words. Watch his reactions, too, as these provide a cue to his response.

- Try not to pretend you've understood him if you haven't. Also resist finishing a sentence or word for him as this could affect his will to communicate.

- Hold conversations on a one-to-one basis, and avoid talking in a crowd.

Coping every day

Even minor tasks can be challenging after a stroke. It can be hard for the person recovering to concentrate, for example on reading or a conversation, or to finish tasks, and he may ask for things to be repeated. Help him to focus on one task at a time, and find ways to make tasks easier. For example, if he finds it hard to scan a page, suggest using a ruler. Make sure, too, that everyday items are kept in the same place to avoid confusion. A wall calendar is helpful, and an established routine for daily tasks gives structure. Allow the person to rest after an activity, and be patient with him as he may be fatigued by the mental effort.

It's important to keep the person stimulated. Simple things, such as planting a window box of lavender or herbs, can stimulate the senses. A lack of stimulation leads to a decline in wellbeing, so any activity, however small, will be of benefit.

Specific perceptual difficulties

Perception is the way the brain interprets the messages it receives from the senses. Vision, hearing, and touch are key to helping us understand our environment and recognize objects. When the brain isn't functioning normally and messages are misunderstood, the person may be unable to carry out a task, or be able to do only part of it. Perceptual problems are not always easy to spot and can be mistaken for something else. For example, problems with visual perception may be interpreted simply as deterioration in eyesight. If you are caring for someone who is recovering from a stroke and you have a particular concern, ask for an assessment from a health professional so that the appropriate action can be taken.

■ **Apraxia** This is the loss or inability to carry out routine tasks even though there is no physical problem. You can help by giving a visual demonstration of a task and clear verbal instructions. Sit beside the person rather than in front and guide his hands to help him complete the task. For example, if he can't get dressed properly, lay his clothes out in the order he would put them on and, if need be, sit on the bed beside him to guide him.

■ **Figure/ground discrimination** This is when a person has difficulty distinguishing objects from their background. Practical solutions are to minimize clutter and label items. Different-coloured labels are helpful, for example a red label on a white fridge handle or on the cooker controls. Highlighting the edge of steps is also useful. Encourage the person to practise recognizing items in a group, for example by sorting coins or laundry, picking out photos, or even finding pictures that you have circled in a magazine.

■ **Agnosia** This is the inability to recognize objects and/or people. Encourage the person you are caring for to practise using the correct names for objects and reinforce their purpose. Be patient and keep things simple. Help with everyday tasks, but don't take over, or his brain won't re-learn tasks.

■ **Right- and left-sided awareness** After a stroke, it is common to lack awareness of one side of the body, although this often improves over time. Encourage the person to use the affected side and approach him and speak to him from that side. Place board games and puzzles in the centre of his vision. If he eats with one hand, get him to place his weaker arm on the table. You could also suggest that he wear a watch that beeps at intervals to remind him to look to his affected side to increase awareness.

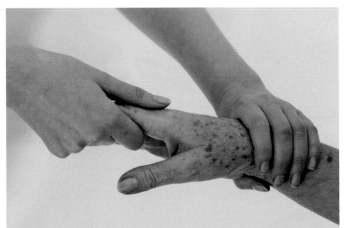

Soothing touch
The sense of touch is important when a person has reduced awareness and ability. If he enjoys it, a hand massage is easy to do. Use a favourite lotion to promote relaxation.

5

MAINTAINING AND AIDING MOBILITY

■ IMPORTANCE OF MOBILITY ■ ASSISTING MOBILITY
■ DEALING WITH FALLS ■ WALKING AIDS
■ EQUIPMENT TO HELP MOVE SOMEONE ■ MOBILITY SCOOTERS
■ WHEELCHAIRS ■ MOBILITY EXERCISES
■ MOBILITY AFTER A STROKE ■ PRESSURE SORES

IMPORTANCE OF MOBILITY

Mobility is important for being able to carry out routine daily activities, such as having a wash in the morning or getting to the toilet, and is vital for maintaining independence. Mobility problems can range from seemingly minor difficulties, such as struggling to get up from a chair, to more serious ones, such as not being able to walk safely unaided. However, each can make it difficult for a person to function with confidence and safety.

Benefits of maintaining mobility

Being active and mobile has a wide range of physical, social, and psychological benefits. It enables a person to maintain independence in everyday activities, which preserves dignity and aids confidence. It also gives the freedom to socialize and participate in activities outside the home.

Physical activity, combined with a healthy diet, can help a person to maintain a good body weight (p.48). Being overweight can make it harder and more painful to move, and the extra weight puts additional stress on the joints. It is also more difficult for the carer to help a heavy person.

Physical activity helps maintain good joint and muscle strength. Even if a person

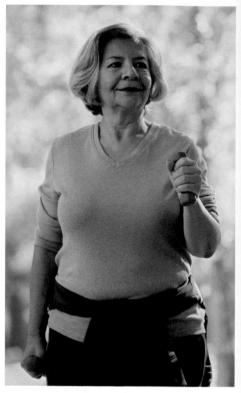

Regular exercise
Walking helps to keep bones and muscles strong and joints flexible. Small weights can be used to increase the benefits to the arms.

CAUSES OF MOBILITY PROBLEMS

Lack of mobility has many different causes, both physical and psychological. Often it is due to a combination of causes.

- Age-related frailty, with conditions such as arthritis, can limit a person's mobility. Without movement, the muscles become weak and the joints become tighter and stiffer.

- Falls affect a third of people over the age of 65 years. Apart from possible injury, they also cause fear and a loss of confidence in walking and remaining active.

- Accidental injury, or perhaps surgery, can lead to pain, with similar psychological effect.

- Mental health conditions such as depression often go alongside physical ill health, reducing further a person's motivation to move or participate in activity.

- Neurological conditions such as Parkinson's disease, stroke, or a head injury will reduce a person's mobility to differing degrees.

- Loss of sight can become a barrier to moving around independently, especially in an unfamiliar environment.

has arthritis, gentle movement or exercise is essential to strengthen the muscles and to maintain each joint's range of movement. Bones are encouraged to lay down more calcium by being used and by having weight put through them, so becoming stronger and less likely to fracture in the event of an accident.

People who are less mobile are at greater risk of pressure sores (p.102) and circulatory problems. However, movement and stretching increases blood flow to the areas of the body involved, improving circulation and reducing the risks of pressure sores developing.

There is a strong link between physical activity and mental health. Staying mobile and participating in exercise can help a person to feel more confident and positive about herself. Being active can also aid relaxation and help a person to sleep when needed, so reducing stress and tiredness.

Suitable activities and exercises

Maintaining mobility doesn't have to involve strenuous exercise; it is as much about being as active as possible. As a carer, you can encourage the person you are looking after to do as much as she can, gradually building up her level of ability and confidence.

Encourage the person you are caring for to take a little physical activity every day. There are many different ways to get exercise, and it is important to find one that the person enjoys. Most activities can be adapted to suit a less able person.

Enjoying the water
For people with stiff joints and restricted movement, swimming or exercising in water can be an enjoyable way of staying active.

■ Gardening is great exercise. Someone who can't stand for too long can sit at a table for smaller tasks, such as sowing seeds or potting up plants, and can use a garden kneeler or seat for work in borders. Long-handled tools that reduce the need for stretching are readily available.

■ Swimming is excellent for keeping joints mobile without putting strain on them and can often be done by people with limited mobiity. The natural buoyancy of the water and the use of flotation aids means they may be able to move their arms and legs more easily than they can out of the water. Some swimming pools have a hoist to allow a less mobile person to enter the water.

■ Dancing is a good group activity and is something you can do with the person you care for. Dancing with a partner can make movement easier, and dance itself can be made simpler or slower if needed.

■ There are specific mobility exercises that target different parts of the body (pp.95–100). They are suitable for the carer as well as the person being cared for. Most can be done while sitting down if necessary.

■ For some people, joining a group is a good incentive, and it is also a good way to meet new people.

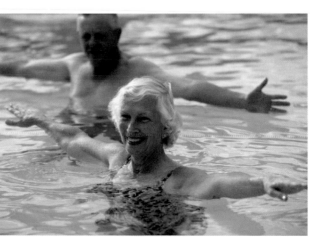

ASSISTING MOBILITY

MAINTAINING AND AIDING MOBILITY

When helping someone with mobility problems, it is very important that you know how to handle the person safely, understand the correct techniques, and know when it may be appropriate to use special equipment to help you.

Professional help

There are a number of care professionals who can advise on regaining, maintaining, and assisting with mobility. An occupational therapist or physiotherapist should be able to assess your situation and provide you with strategies, advice, and information. They can also recommend appropriate adaptations and equipment if necessary, such as raising the height of a bed or chair, or walking aids. Referral to an occupational therapist or physiotherapist is usually made through the GP or hospital doctor of the person you care for.

If you feel that you are unable to provide as much help as is needed, you may need a care assistant (p.22). Your doctor or local social services may be able to advise you.

In the UK, basic mobility equipment that is seen as necessary for maintaining an individual's independence or meeting her care needs is usually supplied through health or social care services.

Handling someone safely

When helping someone whose mobility is compromised, safety for both you and the person you are helping is vital:

■ Make sure you learn the right way to give assistance; ask the occupational therapist or physiotherapist to show you the correct techniques.

■ Prepare the environment. Check that the furniture (the bed /chair/toilet) is a good height, that you have given yourself adequate space, and that you have everything to hand. Make sure that the floor is clear of any trip hazards.

■ Look after your back by maintaining a good posture and keeping close to the person you are helping.

■ Try not to help a person move by putting your arm under her shoulder. This can cause damage to the joint, especially if it is already weak because of age or ill health.

■ Talk to the person you are helping all the time, encouraging her to help you, giving prompts, or just telling her what you are going to do.

■ Give yourself time to carry out any activity; do not rush.

■ Wear non-slippy shoes. The person you are helping should also wear non-slippy shoes if coming to a standing position.

■ Remember that you should not be lifting or taking the weight of the person, just helping her to move. If you are having to take her weight, it is an indicator that you need some mobility equipment (p.88).

LOOKING AFTER YOURSELF

Being a carer can be both physically and emotionally demanding, so it's good for you to be as healthy as possible. When you are busy looking after another person, it can be easy to forget your own needs.

■ Try to plan regular time for yourself at least twice a week if possible. Write it in your diary and prioritize it.

■ The benefits of exercise are the same for everyone. Being physically active will help you to be physically fitter, helping you to sleep and reducing any stress. It can also lift mood.

■ Being part of a group, or being committed to meeting up with a friend, perhaps for a game of tennis, can help you to keep to your routine and makes it a great social activity.

■ If you need to remain at home, consider using an exercise DVD.

HELPING SOMEONE STAND UP

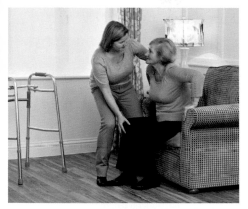

1 Encourage the person to move towards the edge of the chair (or bed); this might be by wriggling or bottom walking (p.112). Position her feet under her knees, with her feet set a little apart. If one leg is stronger than the other, set this foot further back to push up on.

2 Stand to one side but close to the person, sideways on, keeping your feet fairly wide apart. If she is likely to slide forwards off the chair, you can use your outer foot to block her foot. Encourage the person to place her hands on the chair arms on either side, so that she can push herself up. Discourage her from pulling up on walking aids or another piece of furniture.

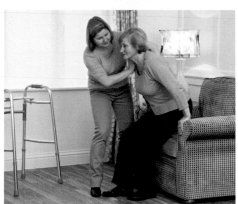

3 Place one of your hands around her back, so that you can provide support as she pushes up. If you need to be at a lower level, remember to bend your knees, not your back. Place your other hand gently at the front of the shoulder closest to you. This hand is just giving the feeling of security and helping her to retain her balance as she stands.

4 You may find it helpful to count to three, with the person rocking gently forwards on each count, using the momentum to stand fully on "three". Encourage her to lean right forwards, "nose over toes" as she lifts from the chair and then pushes up, using her leg muscles to stand.

5 Once she is standing, make sure she has her balance. You can then hand over any walking aid that is needed.

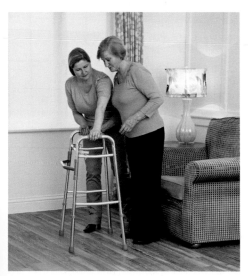

HELPING SOMEONE SIT DOWN

If you need to help a person sit down you can almost reverse the process of standing up.

- Encourage her to get as close to the chair (or bed) as possible before sitting down. She should feel the chair on the backs of her legs

- Make sure she puts her hands back to the chair before sitting down, so she can control herself as she lowers her body weight.

- Your position should be the same as for helping her stand up, giving support around the back but not taking her weight.

» ASSISTING MOBILITY

Helping a person walk

Before you start helping someone walk, make sure she feels well enough. Anyone who feels dizzy, unwell, or weaker than usual should not try to walk.

If a person needs a walking aid (p.86), make sure it is to hand, and that it is the right height and in good condition.

If the person can walk without any aids but still needs a little support, then you can steady her by standing close to her side and giving support under her elbow with one hand, or perhaps putting an arm around her back. Hold her other hand, palm to palm.

(p.86)

HELPING SOMEONE WITH IMPAIRED VISION

A person with poor vision may at times need help to move in an unfamiliar environment. Always ask how she would like to be guided.

- Stand next to the person on whichever side she wants you to be.

- Usually the person will grasp your arm just above the elbow. Keep your upper arm straight, held close to the side of your body.

- The person will be able to walk just a little behind you, feeling your body move, turn, or change height as you lead her.

- Slow down as you approach doors, steps, and the like, describing them clearly.

- When approaching steps with a hand rail, let the person be on the side with the rail.

- If you have to swap sides, ask the person to stand still while you move and guide her hand to the rail.

- For detailed advice on guiding someone with impaired vision, see the website of the Royal National Institute of Blind People (RNIB, p.214).

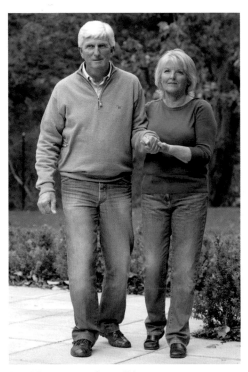

Providing support for walking
Stand next to the person and support under his elbow with one hand. Hold his other hand, with your palm on his palm.

Helping a person up and down stairs

It is important that you take your time when helping someone on the stairs. Ensure the stairs are well lit and that there are no trip hazards such as loose carpets. If possible, install a banister rail on both sides for the full length of the stairs. If space allows, you can keep a suitable chair at the top or bottom of each flight of stairs to rest upon.

Never stand immediately behind or in front of the person in case she falls and knocks you down, and make sure she has a good grip of the banister rail(s). If there is only one rail for her to hold, stand on the side without a rail.

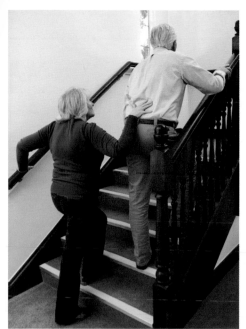

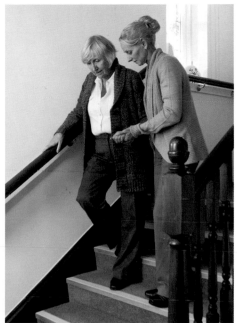

Climbing stairs
Stand slightly behind and to the side of the person. Gently support his back with your nearest hand (or use a transfer belt). Use your other hand to steady yourself or hold the rail on your side if one is present. If he has one side stronger than the other, encourage him to step up with the stronger leg first, then bring the second leg up to the same step. Repeat, one step at a time, until you reach the top.

Descending stairs
Make sure the person has a good grip of the banister rail(s). If there is only one rail for her to hold, you can stand on the other side and support her arm. If she has one side stronger than the other, encourage her to step down with the weaker leg first, then bring the second leg down to the same step. If she feels she is going to fall, don't try to support her weight, but help her to sit down on the stairs.

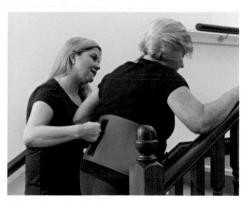

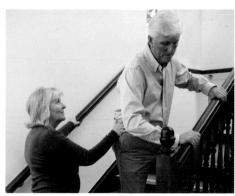

Using a transfer belt
A transfer belt, which goes around the person's waist, can be used to provide support.

Holding with two hands
If the person needs to hold a single rail with both hands, he can take each step sideways on.

DEALING WITH FALLS

Falls are common in elderly people, and you need to know how to help if someone starts to fall or if a person has fallen.

CONTROLLING A FALL

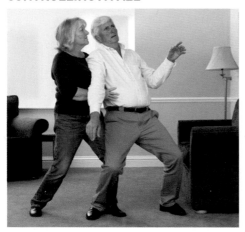

1 If there is time, try to get behind the person with your arms around his upper body. Do not try to take his weight in your arms. Brace your legs wide apart and bend your knees, keeping your back straight.

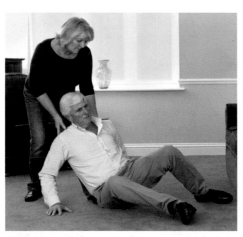

2 Allow him to slide down your body onto the floor. If you can, guide him away from the sharp corners of furniture or hard objects, protecting his head as much as you can.

What to do if someone starts to fall

If someone falls, it can be your immediate response to try to stop her, but this can be very dangerous for you. If you are standing close to the person you are helping and she begins to feel dizzy, or you feel her begin to fall, don't try to stop the fall, but guide her down onto a soft chair or to the floor so that the fall has less impact.

However, falls can happen very quickly and it is not always possible to control another person as she falls. If you cannot get behind a person, you may be able to steer her to a nearby wall, so that she slides down the wall.

What to do if someone has fallen

If you have witnessed a fall, or found someone who has fallen, check if she is hurt or unwell. If the person shows any signs of serious injury or shock, first deal with this (pp.174–189). Do not move the person, other than to ensure she can breathe. Call an ambulance. If you know

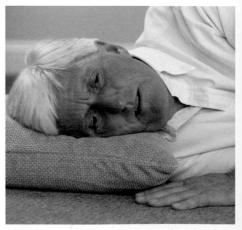

3 Once he is safely on the floor, help him into a comfortable position and place a cushion under his head. Let him rest until he feels ready to get up.

the person has diabetes, you may need to give extra care (see panel, p.151).

If the person has no pain or injury, see if she can move carefully and slowly. If so, you can help her to pull herself up to standing. Sometimes a person can fall into a very awkward position or place that she cannot move out of, or be moved out of by you. In this situation, call an ambulance.

HELPING A PERSON WHO HAS FALLEN AND IS ABLE TO MOVE

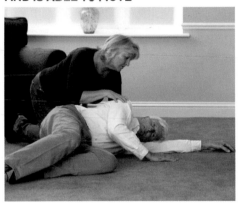

1 Encourage the person to roll onto his side, and see if he can push himself up to side-sitting. You may need to kneel or sit on the floor alongside to help him, but make sure that you do not strain yourself.

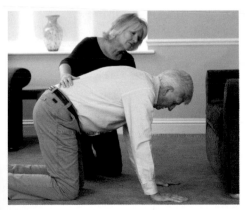

2 Encourage him to raise himself onto his hands and knees so that he is in a crawling position, if possible.

CAUSES OF FALLING

Possible causes for falls in elderly people include the following.

- Age-related stiffness of joints and weaker muscles. Regular exercise to keep muscles and joints strong is important.
- Impaired vision. When caring for someone with poor vision, it is especially important to keep rooms uncluttered.
- Not eating and drinking enough due to dementia. This can lead to falls because the body is not getting enough hydration or energy. There are steps you can take to help someone with dementia eat better (p.56).
- Underlying medical conditions such as a heart problem or a neurological condition like Parkinson's disease or stroke.
- The side effects of some medications, or taking multiple medicines. If a person experiences dizziness or unusual sleepiness when she takes her medicines, discuss this with her doctor.
- Use of sleeping pills. These can cause drowsiness or unsteadiness the next day, increasing the risk of falls. Sleeping pills should only be used as a last resort (p.106).

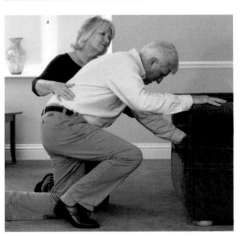

3 If he is able, he can crawl towards a chair (you may need to move one closer to him). Once close enough, he can place his hands on the chair for support as he raises himself from the floor onto one knee. When very close to the seat of the chair, he can turn around slowly and carefully to sit on the chair.

WALKING AIDS

Anyone with mobility problems should be seen by a physiotherapist to be assessed and, if required, provided with a walking aid. If a person has been admitted to hospital, the assessment will be made there. If not, the person's GP can refer her.

Choice of walking aid

Walking aids are designed to take some of the weight that the legs would otherwise bear when walking. The choice of walking aid is governed by the person's level of mobility, how safely she is able to move around, and any difficulty she may have in gripping an aid.

The main types of aid are walking sticks, elbow crutches, and walking frames. Walking sticks can help with stability but are only suitable if the person has a fairly stable and safe gait. As weight is taken through the hand, their use may be limited by conditions such as arthritis. Elbow crutches give slightly better stability, while

walking frames are the most stable type of walking aid and may be the safest option if a person is very wobbly. A container (caddy) can be attached to the front of many frames, enabling small items to be transported.

GETTING THE RIGHT HEIGHT

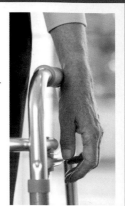

It is important for the height of a walking stick or frame to be adjusted for the person using it. When the person stands and holds her arm straight down, the walking stick or the handles of the frame should come up to the sharp bone at the side of the wrist. The therapist who issued the aid will ensure the correct fit.

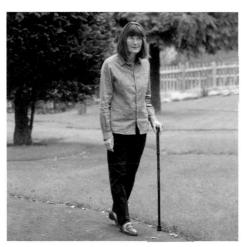

Using a walking stick
A single walking stick should be held on the side of the stronger leg, and moved forwards at the same time as the weaker leg.

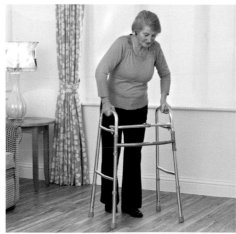

Using a walking frame
The frame should be placed one step ahead. The person then walks towards it, using the weaker leg first, followed by the other leg.

TYPES OF WALKING AID

WALKING AID	DESCRIPTION
Walking sticks	■ Only suitable if a person has a fairly stable, safe gait. ■ Available with different handles: the T-handle (far right) is the most common and suits a wide range of people. The crook handle (near right) can be hard to grasp and is not suitable for people who need to put a lot of weight on the stick.
Elbow crutches	■ Have handles for the person to hold and a band that encircles the forearm. ■ Will support a person like a walking stick, but give better forearm support, increasing balance and stability.
Standard walking frame	■ The most common type of walking frame has moulded plastic or foam rubber handgrips and four points of contact with the floor, enabling a person to lean onto the frame.
Rollator frame	■ Similar to the standard frame, but the front two points of contact have small wheels, which allows the person to push the frame forwards rather than lift it. ■ Not suitable for use outside as the wheels may get caught in rough surfaces.
Three-wheeled walker	■ Has a single wheel at the front and one either side. ■ Usually has lockable brakes, and the two sides fold together for ease of storage or transport. ■ Is safe to use outside. ■ Is easier to move than a rollator, so the person needs to be stable enough to control her own speed.
Trolley	■ Has four wheels, a pushing handle at one end, and two melamine-covered shelves (p.37). ■ Provides support and stability for walking, while enabling transport of small items such as a meal or a cup of tea.
Gutter frame	■ Specialized walking frame for those who cannot put any weight through their hands, perhaps due to severe arthritis. ■ To use the frame, the person leans her forearms into gutters attached to the frame and holds onto upright grips at the front of the gutter on each side. ■ Is a large piece of equipment, and consideration should be given to the space available in the home to use the frame safely.

EQUIPMENT TO HELP MOVE SOMEONE

A wide range of equipment is available for helping to move someone, and technological advances are being made all the time. Equipment can range from simple items that provide some support during moving, such as a transfer belt, to complex items such as hoists that take the full weight of a person.

TYPES OF EQUIPMENT

EQUIPMENT	PURPOSE
Transfer belt	■ Goes around the person's waist and gives the carer a secure grip to help the person when she is moving, for example going up or down stairs (p.83).
Turntable disc	■ An easily portable disc that allows someone to be turned easily. ■ The person stands on the disc and can then be swivelled round to face in a different direction, for example when getting out of a car.
Transfer board	■ A flat, low-friction board that allows a person to slide from one surface to another. ■ There are different types: the one shown right is specially for transfer to toilet or commode (see also opposite).
Turner	■ Helps a carer to move a seated person from one surface to another, such as a wheelchair to a bed, but is only suitable for people who can maintain a standing position. ■ The turner is adjusted so that the person's knees are against the knee pads and she is able to grasp the handles to pull up to standing. The carer then rotates the turner until the new surface is behind the person; she can then lower herself down.
Swivel seat cushion	■ Enables a person to rotate on a surface while seated. ■ Can be useful when getting in and out of cars.
Slide sheet	■ A two-layered piece of very low-friction material that enables a person to be slid along a surface, such as a bed (p.115), or transferred from one surface to another.
Hoist	■ A large piece of equipment that can mechanically lift a person from one surface to another using a sling (p.90). ■ It may be advisable for two people to operate a hoist.

Training and safely

It's important that you know how to use each piece of equipment and that you follow the correct safety procedures, as explained by the physiotherapist or occupational therapist.

■ Make sure that the equipment is in good condition and not worn or damaged.

■ If two carers are recommended for using a piece of equipment, make sure that someone else is available to help you.

■ Check there is enough space for both the equipment and the carer(s).

■ Explain to the person you are helping how the equipment works and what will happen during the move.

■ If, during the move, the person feels any pain or anxiety, stop immediately.

■ If you had to move any furniture out of the way, it is important to return it to its original position so that the person knows where things are and is reassured by her familiar environment.

USING A TRANSFER BOARD

1 To move from a bed to a chair using a transfer board, the person must first be sitting on the edge of the bed, with the chair positioned alongside at 90 degrees to the bed.

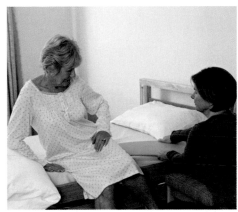

2 The person leans away while one end of the board is carefully tucked under her buttocks. The other end of the board must reach part way across the seat of the chair.

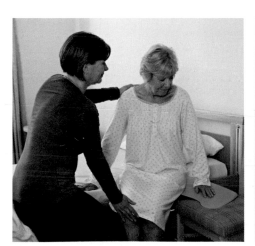

3 The person places the hand nearest the chair flat on the board, being careful not to curl her fingers under it. Using her upper limb strength, she starts to slide herself along the board towards the chair.

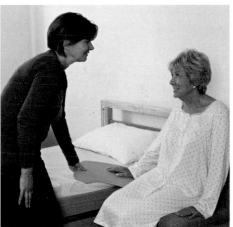

4 She continues to edge herself along the board towards the chair until she is fully across and in the chair. She will need to lean away from the transfer board as it is removed from under her buttocks.

» EQUIPMENT TO HELP MOVE SOMEONE

Types of hoist

When a person becomes unable to stand or to be moved using a transfer board, a health professional may suggest a hoist as an alternative way of moving her.

There are a number of kinds of hoist. When choosing one, the person's condition, lifestyle, and wishes, as well as the carer's ability and environmental factors, need to be considered. Most people in their own homes are provided with a standard mobile, battery-powered hoist, with a sling-lifting mechanism. If required, there are alternatives such as ceiling-track hoists. Slings come in different designs and sizes.

Lifting someone with a hoist
When raising the hoist, stay close to the person and provide encouragement and reassurance to ease any anxieties she may have.

The correct sling must be used – this depends on the size of the person being hoisted and the purpose of lifting her, for example for straightforward transfers or perhaps for going to the toilet.

The hoist should be serviced regularly and the sling checked. The hoist provider should be able to advise you on this.

Using a hoist safely

Although a hoist does all the lifting for you, it is still quite a slow and complex process and sometimes needs two people to be completely safe. If you are going to be involved in the hoisting process, ensure that you receive proper training. Use the following checklist to remind yourself of the correct procedure.

- Have everything that is needed to hand.
- Make sure the area is clear and free from hazards; the hoist should be out of the way until you have fitted the sling.
- Fit the sling under the person in the correct position.
- Bring in the hoist so that the bar attached to the lifting mechanism is over the person's chest.
- Lower the hoist, being careful not to knock the person with the bar.
- Attach the sling securely.
- Partially raise the hoist, so the sling can be checked, and adjusted if necessary.
- Fully raise the hoist.
- Move the person into her new position over the chair (or bed or commode).
- As the hoist is lowered, position the person back into the chair.
- Disconnect the sling from the hoist.
- Move the hoist out of the way.
- Carefully remove the sling from under the person.

MOBILITY SCOOTERS

A mobility scooter can enable someone to get around with relative ease. There are three basic types of scooter. The smallest, sometimes called miniscooters, are more suited to indoor use. Mid-size scooters can be used outside but are only suitable for use on pavements or footpaths. Larger, slightly faster, powered vehicles can be driven on the road as long as legal regulations are met (see panel, right).

Choosing a scooter

Information about purchasing a scooter in the UK is available from the Disabled Living Foundation (p.214). The following factors should be considered:

- Is the person using the scooter fit enough to do so? Make sure she doesn't have any problems with her sight, hearing, or any other medical condition that might make her unsafe.
- Is the scooter needed for indoor and/or outdoor use? Be aware of legal regulations for vehicles that might be used on the road.
- Consider any restrictions there might be in or near the person's home, such as door or gate widths.

- Consider where the scooter will be securely stored.
- The scooter battery will need recharging, usually every day. Is there a power point nearby, or can you carry the battery to a suitable power point?
- The scooter will have an initial purchase cost, but also ongoing maintenance costs. Can these be maintained?
- Scooters can have different features, such as swivel seating. Before choosing, it is advisable to look at and try some of the options available.

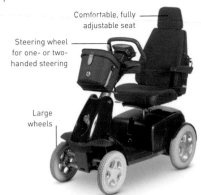

Basket for transporting items

Lifting handle for carrying when folded up

Anti-tip wheels

Comfortable, fully adjustable seat

Steering wheel for one- or two-handed steering

Large wheels

Miniscooter
The smallest type of scooter, mainly for indoor use, can only go short distances, but is small enough to be folded into a car boot.

Road-legal mobility scooter
More powerful scooters can be driven on roads at up to 12.8kph (8mph). Use on dual carriageways, though legal, is not recommended.

WHEELCHAIRS

MAINTAINING AND AIDING MOBILITY

The provision of wheelchairs by the NHS in the UK is limited. Before being offered one, a person needs to undergo an assessment to determine eligibility. Referral is usually through an occupational therapist or the person's doctor.

Wheelchairs may be hired from several charities and other organizations (p.214), General advice is available from hospital or community occupational therapy services.

Choice of wheelchair

Wheelchairs are of three main types: self-propelled, those designed to be pushed solely by an attendant, and electric. Most manual wheelchairs have the brake controls at the level of the wheels, but some also have them on the handlebars, making it easier for the carer.

The choice of wheelchair depends on a person's individual's needs. Just because a wheelchair user relies on an attendant to push her does not necessarily mean that an attendant-propelled chair is the best choice. If she is a full-time wheelchair user, a self-propelled type of wheelchair may be more suitable as it has larger wheels and is more robust and manoeuvrable than an attendant-propelled chair.

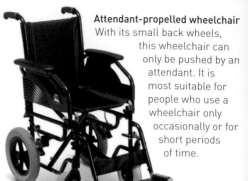

Attendant-propelled wheelchair
With its small back wheels, this wheelchair can only be pushed by an attendant. It is most suitable for people who use a wheelchair only occasionally or for short periods of time.

Electric wheelchairs may be considered by people who are unable to manoeuvre a chair on their own, for example due to pain or fatigue. There are different types available, depending on whether they are for indoor use only, for use on pavements, or capable of being used on the road (Class 3). The same legal requirements apply to Class 3 wheelchairs as to Class 3 mobility scooters (p.91). An electric wheelchair will need to be stored in a secure and waterproof place close to a power point so that the batteries can be charged.

Fit and comfort

Once the decision about type of wheelchair has been made, you need to make sure that the seat is wide enough. You should be able to get your hands down the side of the person's thighs when she is sitting in the chair. If the chair is too tight against her legs, there is a risk of skin damage or pressure sores (p.102).

It is important that there is a cushion for the person to sit on. For someone who has the ability to move within the chair and who has good skin condition on her bottom and over the lower back, a standard 5cm (2in) sponge cushion is adequate. For someone

Self-propelled wheelchair
This chair has large back wheels and can be propelled by the user or an attendant. It is more manoeuvrable than an attendant-propelled chair.

who is at risk of, or already has, pressure sores a suitable pressure-relieving cushion should be used.

Getting in an out of a wheelchair
Make sure that the brakes are applied and that the footplates are tilted up and swung out of the way as the person gets in or out of the chair. If she can manage to do this independently, you can hold the chair from behind to give it more stability.

If she needs help to get in or out of the chair, the method is the same as for standing up and sitting down from a bed or chair (p.81). If she is unable to stand to move into the chair, she may be able to slide into it using a transfer board (p.89).

Pushing a wheelchair
When pushing someone in a wheelchair, make sure she sits right to the back of the chair. If she is at any risk of falling out of the chair, use a lap strap. Always use the footplates when you move to protect the person's feet.

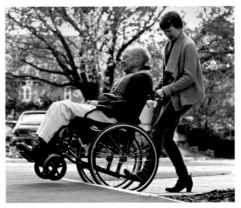

Negotiating a kerb
If you have to go up or down a kerb, approach it straight on. Tilt the chair backwards by pushing down on the tipping lever with your foot. Don't overtilt the chair. If you need to go down a kerb, it is easier and safer to go down backwards.

When pushing a wheelchair outside, try to stay off the road, sticking to smooth, level surfaces as far as possible. If you need to cross a road, try to use dropped kerbs and pedestrian crossings. If you have to stop on a slope, remember to apply the brakes. Always move slowly and carefully, telling the person in the chair what you are doing. If the wheelchair is self-propelling, ask the person to help you.

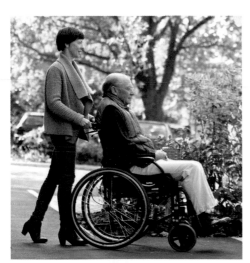

Pushing a wheelchair
It is quite hard work to push a wheelchair. You need to be aware of your posture at all times and try to keep your back straight.

WHEELCHAIR MAINTENANCE

The wheelchair user or carer should check the wheelchair regularly, to keep it safe and easy to use. If you spot any problems, talk to the wheelchair provider. Regularly check that:

- Brakes are secure when applied.
- Tyres are pumped up.
- The framework and the fabric are in good condition and the wheelchair is clean.
- Nuts and bolts are tight.
- Footplates and armrests can be released and put back easily.
- The wheelchair opens and closes easily.

›› WHEELCHAIRS

FOLDING A WHEELCHAIR INTO A CAR BOOT

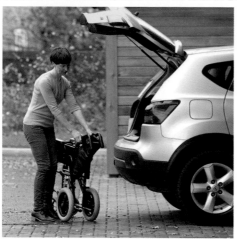

1 If possible, first reduce the weight of the chair by taking off all the removable parts. Apply the brakes to lock the wheels. Fold the wheelchair by pulling upwards on the middle of the seat (or using the grab strap, if present). If possible, fold down the back.

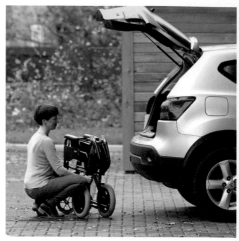

2 Standing to the side of the wheelchair, bend your knees as you squat down, taking care to keep your back straight. Grab the frame with both hands, with one hand positioned just above the front wheel and the other just above the back wheel.

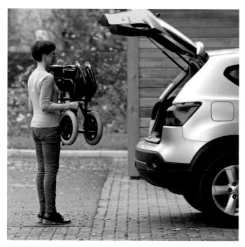

3 Using your leg muscles to do the work and keeping your back straight, lift the wheelchair straight up against your hips.

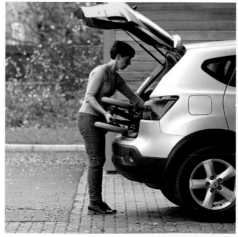

4 Pivot the bottom of the chair to waist height, wheels towards the boot, and slide the chair into the boot.

MOBILITY EXERCISES

Exercise is good for you and the person for whom you are caring. The following is advice that is applicable to both of you. Remember to prepare yourselves and start exercising carefully. Make sure that clothes and shoes are appropriate. Drink plenty of water. Always warm up with some gentle activity and stretching.

It is good to get your heart and your breathing to speed up a little, but if at any time you or the person you are caring for feel faint, nauseous, unusually breathless, or in pain, stop the exercise. If the symptoms don't go away with rest, contact a doctor for advice. If you or the person

have had surgery or have injured any part of the body, take medical advice to know when it is safe to start exercising and then start very gently, slowly building up the amount that is done. The same rule applies if you or the person hasn't exercised for a long time.

Many of these exercises can be done while seated. Select the ones that are best suited to you or the person you are caring for. Do a little to begin with, then a little more each time. You or she might like some music on in the background to give some rhythm to do the exercises to. Try to breathe evenly and easily. Breathe in as you stretch, and breathe out as you relax.

SHOULDER ROTATIONS

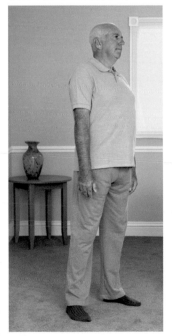
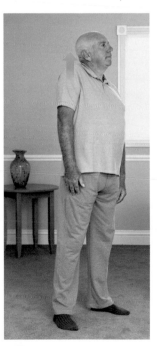
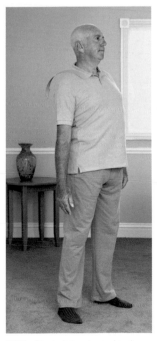

1 Stand or sit up as straight as possible, with your legs slightly apart, stretching but not arching your back, with your arms down by your sides.

2 Lift one shoulder up towards your ear, trying to keep the rest of your body still and your arms relaxed as you do the movement.

3 Circle it backwards, down and round to the front. Repeat 6 times slowly and smoothly, then swap to the other shoulder and repeat.

95

» MOBILITY EXERCISES

ARM ROTATIONS

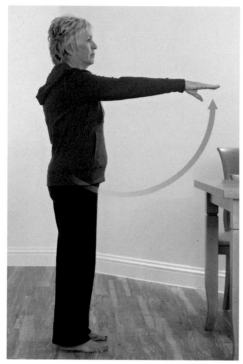

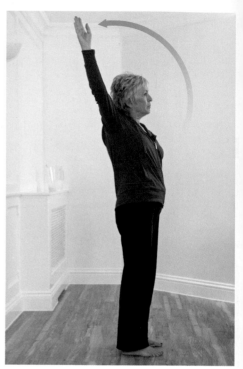

1 Stand or sit up as straight as possible, stretching but not arching your back. Gently lift one arm up in front of you, keeping the elbow as straight as possible.

2 Continue to lift it up above your head and then gently back down behind you. Repeat the circling movement six times, then swap to the other arm and repeat.

EXERCISING IN A CHAIR

Many exercises can be done while sitting in a chair. This means they can be carried out even by people with restricted mobility or those who are unable to stand for long, for example due to balance problems or pain. Chair-based exercises avoid impact on joints and limit energy expenditure to the specific exercise being done. Make sure the chair used for exercising fits properly, and is comfortable and supportive. The exercises can also be done in a wheelchair.

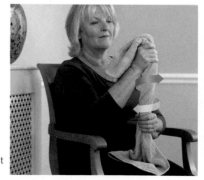

Wrist strengthener
Roll or fold up a towel (or tights or exercise band). Grasp the towel with both hands, squeeze hard, then twist by bringing the elbows in close to your body. Hold for a count of five, then relax for a few seconds. Repeat eight times.

NECK STRETCH

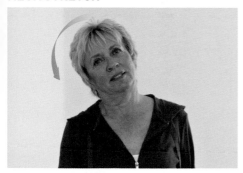 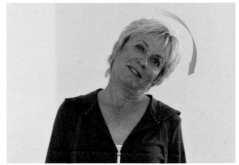

1 Stand or sit up as straight as possible, stretching but not arching your back. Imagine the top of your head stretched up, with your chin tucked in. Keep your shoulders down. Looking forwards, lean your head to one side. Try to hold the stretch for a slow count of three.

2 Bring your head back to the centre. Once again, imagine the top of your head being stretched up, with your chin tucked in. Lean your head to the other side and hold the stretch for a slow count of three. Repeat the movement, leaning each way six times.

SIDEWAYS LEAN

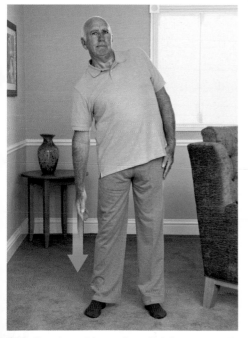 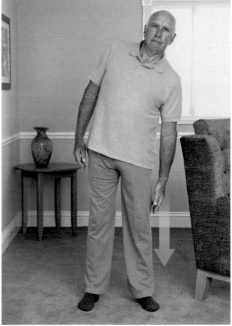

1 Stand up with your feet slightly apart, or sit straight in your chair. Rest your hands on your hips if possible. Gently lean sideways. Try to hold the stretch for a slow count of three.

2 Straighten up to your starting position, then lean to the other side and hold the stretch for a slow count of three. Repeat the movement, leaning each way six times.

» MOBILITY EXERCISES

CHEST STRETCH

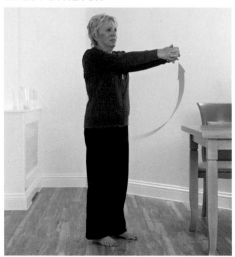

1 Stand up with your feet slightly apart, or sit straight in your chair, stretching but not arching your back. Lift your arms up in front of you and grip one hand with the other, perhaps interlinking your fingers.

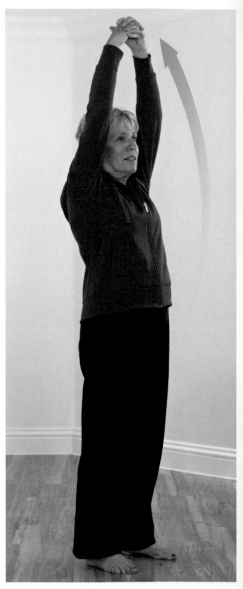

USING SMALL WEIGHTS

Some people use small weights to exercise their arms. This can be done by someone sitting down. If you don't have weights, you can always fill some small water bottles to use.

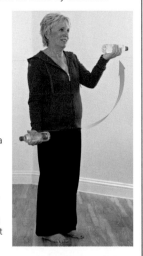

Biceps curl
Stand or sit with your feet slightly apart, palms facing forwards, a weight in each hand. Lift one weight up slowly by bending your elbow. Lower the weight, then lift the weight on the other side. Repeat six times.

2 Slowly raise both your arms up above your head, trying to keep your elbows as straight as possible. Try to hold the stretch for a slow count of three, then lower your arms again. Repeat the movement six times.

SQUATS

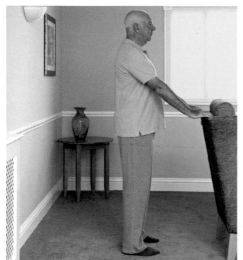

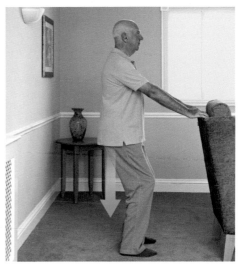

1 Not everyone can do squats, so don't push yourself. Use a stable piece of furniture (such as the back of an armchair) if you need extra support. Holding onto your support, stand with your feet quite wide apart.

2 Gently bend at the knees and lower your upper body, keeping your back as straight as possible, head looking forwards. Only go down as far as it is comfortable. Repeat the movement five times to start with, if possible. Each time you exercise, do one extra squat until you can do 10.

TOP TURNS

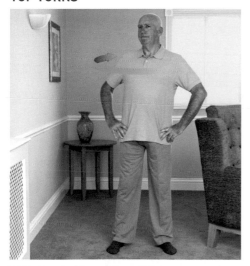

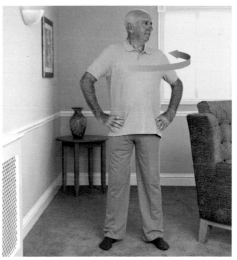

1 Stand with your feet slightly apart, or sit straight in your chair. Rest your hands on your hips if possible. Try to keep your hips facing forwards as you gently rotate your upper body towards one side. Hold the stretch for a slow count of three.

2 Turn back to centre. Then gently rotate your upper body to the other side and hold the stretch for a slow count of three. Repeat the entire sequence, turning one way and then the other, for a total of six times.

» MOBILITY EXERCISES

MARCHING ON THE SPOT

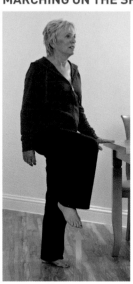

1 Stand or sit up as straight as possible. You may need to support yourself on the back of a chair or other piece of furniture. Begin marching on the spot by bending one knee to lift your foot off the floor.

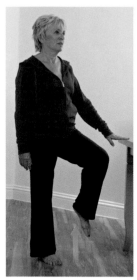

2 Replace your foot on the floor, and lift up the other foot as you bend your knee. Continue to march on the spot, lifting one foot then the other, counting a regular rhythm to yourself. Start by marching for just a short period, building up over time. If you get very breathless, or your heart is pumping very strongly, stop and rest.

LEG RAISERS

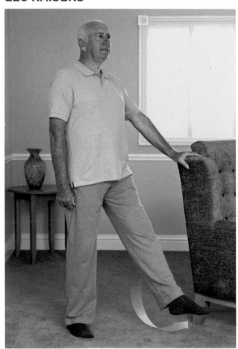

1 Stand sideways on to a supporting chair. Make sure you are safe balancing on one leg, holding the chair. Gently raise the leg nearest the chair out in front of you, trying to keep your knee as straight as possible. Hold the stretch for a slow count of three, then lower your leg again. Repeat the movement six times.

2 Turn so that your other leg is nearest the supporting chair and repeat the movement six times with this leg. If you are in a chair, you can lift alternate legs out in front of you.

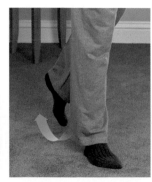

3 If you are able to, you can do the exercise described in Steps 1 and 2, but this time stretching each leg out behind you.

MOBILITY AFTER A STROKE

A stroke is a serious condition that occurs when blood supply to part of the brain is cut off, and it can result in reduced movement on one side of the body. There is often a pattern to the way movement is affected after a stroke. Initially, the limbs are floppy; more normal muscle tone and movement then returns, to be followed by an increase in muscle tone. Increased muscle tone may result in spasticity – uncontrollable tightening of muscles – causing abnormal positioning of limbs.

Sometimes a person who has had a stroke does not regain full use of the limbs. However, with the help of therapists, she can learn to adapt activities or learn new ways to manage them.

Therapy after a stroke

Therapists will first work with the person to help her regain movement in the muscles nearest the main trunk of the body so that she is able to roll, sit unaided, and perhaps crawl. Work will then begin on the muscles of the legs, arms, hands, and feet. They will aim to help the person eventually regain the ability to stand and to walk, along with fine movements such as finger grip.

The therapists will try to prevent muscle spasticity by moving and positioning the person to oppose the pattern that the spasticity is causing. Such treatment is important as spasticity can lead to permanent tightening of the muscles and joints, causing pain and a loss of mobility.

How you can help

The amount of assistance a person will require depends on how much effect the stroke has had. As a carer, you should receive training from a therapist before you try to help the person you are caring for.

> ### HELPING AFTER A STROKE
>
> There are several guiding principles when helping a person who has lost mobility after a stroke:
>
> - Normality in terms of positioning and movement.
> - Prevention of spasticity through stretching of muscles and good positioning while at rest.
> - Protection of any limb or part of the body that remains floppy or numb.

You can help the person to maintain a normal position with good posture even while she is sitting. She should be able to sit with her hips and knees at 90 degrees, with her feet flat on the floor. Make sure her arms are supported on the arms of the chair, in her lap, or on top of a cushion or pillow to encourage her fingers to be straight, not curled.

If you are helping or supervising a person to walk after a stroke, stand on the affected weaker side and slightly behind her. If she is fairly stable, gently support her with your hands placed on each side of her hips below the waist. If she needs more support, use a transfer belt (p.889). If she has a floppy arm, protect it by supporting the arm lightly or by using a sling.

If the person uses a stick, this is held in the stronger arm. If she is able to grip with both hands, she may use a frame. In each case, she should move the walking aid one step's length ahead and then take one step forwards. Encourage her to take her time and to keep her steps quite small.

Sometimes speech and understanding can be affected by a stroke. A speech and language therapist can advise you how best to communicate with the person (p.74).

PRESSURE SORES

Pressure sores are skin ulcers caused by compression and consequent disruption of blood supply to the area. They often occur in people with limited mobility who find it difficult to change position and so continually put weight on the same areas. Pressure sores develop on parts of the body that take the most pressure when a person sits or lies down, especially where there are bony prominences.

The risk of developing pressure sores is higher in people who are very thin, have poor nutritional and fluid intake, poor circulation, or reduced sensation. People with incontinence are also at higher risk, due to dampness of skin.

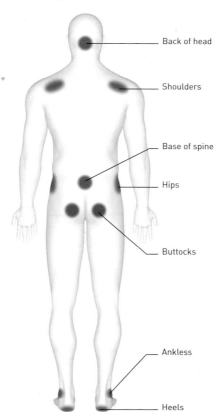

Back of head

Shoulders

Base of spine

Hips

Buttocks

Ankless

Heels

Monitoring the skin

If the person you are caring for has reduced mobility, you will need to monitor her body for potential pressure areas. If pressure sores are caught early, they are much easier to treat and will heal better. Ask the person to tell you if she gets any tender areas of skin, and be on the lookout for any red areas. If preventive steps (below) are not taken at this stage, a pressure sore may develop: the skin becomes painful and discoloured, and eventually breaks down to form an ulcer.

If a pressure sore starts to form, it is important that you contact the person's doctor as soon as possible. Left untreated, a pressure sore will get bigger and deeper and may become infected.

Prevention

Make sure the person's skin is kept as clean as dry as possible, especially if she suffers from incontinence combined with poor mobility. Encourage her to maintain a healthy protein- and vitamin-rich diet and to drink plenty of water. She should wear loose-fitting clothing, without hard or bulky seams. Use natural fibre bedding and keep it wrinkle-free.

If the person is able to walk, she should move at least once an hour. If in a chair, leaning to alternate sides to take the pressure off each buttock can help and should be done once or twice an hour. If she is unable to move, you will need to help her. This might be changing her position in bed (p.112), alternating between side-lying and lying on her back. It is very important

Common sites for pressure sores
Pressure sores develop over bony prominences of the body, and most commonly occur at the sites indicated on the diagram.

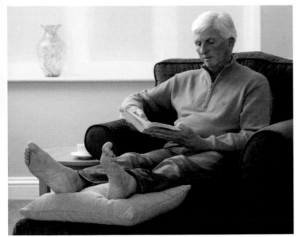

Taking the pressure off
For people who sit for long periods, raising the legs on a footstool periodically can help to redistribute pressure. Place a pillow under all of the lower leg to avoid pressure on the heel.

to help the person stay in the best position. The cushions and mattresses are made of different materials, with differing degrees of pressure relief. Other pressure-relieving equipment includes bed cradles (p.111), which support the weight of bedclothes to relieve pressure, and fleece or gel bootees worn to protect the heels and ankles.

A health professional, such as a district nurse or occupational therapist, will be able to give advice on the most appropriate cushions, mattress, or other pressure-relieving equipment if a pressure area begins to develop.

to avoid shearing the skin if you are helping a person to move.

Positioning a person is also important. Don't let her slouch down in a chair when seated as this causes increased pressure at the base of the spine. Encourage her to sit with good posture, with a right angle of 90 degrees at the knees and hips. If using a footstool, she should not rest all the weight of the leg on the heel; to avoid this, place a pillow under the whole of the lower leg. If a person has a very bony spine or shoulders, use pillows to create support around her back, spreading the weight as she lies back in bed or leans against the back of a chair.

Pressure-relieving equipment

Some pressure-relieving cushions and mattresses aim to mould around the shape of the person to redistribute the pressure over a greater surface area; others mechanically vary the pressure beneath the individual, so reducing the duration of the pressure at any one point (p.111). Cushions are sometimes moulded

Treatment

The doctor is likely to refer a person who is developing a pressure sore to the district nurses. They will treat the wound, most importantly by keeping the area clean and dry. If there is existing infection, antibiotics will be given.

The sore may be covered with a dressing that does not stick to the affected area. The type of dressing used depends on the seriousness of the sore, ranging from simple gauze to one that actively promotes healing.

The nurses may need to remove dead tissue from an open sore, a procedure known as debridement. There are a number of ways that this is done, and the nurse will discuss the options with you and the person being cared for.

For a deeper, more extensive sore, surgery may be required to clean the wound and then close it, sometimes using tissue from a nearby area of the body.

6

COMFORT IN BED

■ REST AND SLEEP ■ BEDS AND BEDDING
■ EQUIPMENT TO AID COMFORT ■ MOBILITY IN BED

REST AND SLEEP

Most people need between six and nine hours sleep per night. The pattern of sleeping changes with age, with older people tending to spend more time in lighter sleep and to wake up more often at night than younger people.

Why sleep is important

Sleep is important for wellbeing in numerous ways. Poor sleep at night will make the person sleepy during the day, increasing the risk of falls and other accidents. It can make the person more irritable, stressed, and unable to concentrate, making learning more difficult and memory poorer. The person's metabolism and immune system can become disrupted as a result of poor sleep, leading to weight gain and illness.

If sleep becomes a real problem, contact the person's doctor, who can help to identify any underlying health problems that might be interfering with sleep. Sleeping tablets should be a last resort and

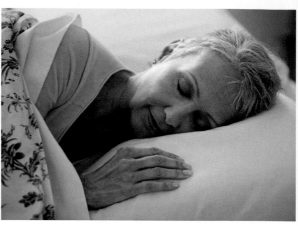

A good night's sleep
Getting enough sleep is vital for physical and mental wellbeing. A peaceful environment and a comfortable bed help ensure a good night's sleep.

ideally not used in the long term. Even with short-term use, It is easy to become dependent on them. In addition to the risk of dependency, sleeping tablets can have unwanted side effects the next day, causing unsteadiness and a drowsy feeling. These side effects are more common in elderly people and increase the risk of falls.

SLEEPING PATTERNS

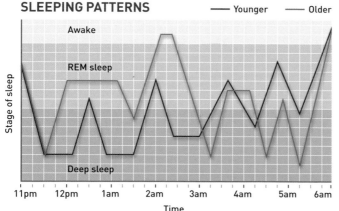

Sleeping patterns
Generally, older people spend less time in deep sleep than those who are younger. Older people typically have more periods of REM (rapid eye movement) sleep, which is associated with greater brain activity than NREM (non-rapid eye movement), or deep, sleep when brain waves slow down and a person is hard to wake.

Common reasons for poor sleep

One of the most common causes of disturbed sleep is the need to get up to pass urine (nocturia), and this is likely to increase with age. For an elderly person, this increases the risk of night-time falls.

Older people are more likely to experience physical discomfort, such as aching limbs or stiff joints, that can keep them awake. A bed or bedding that is uncomfortable can exacerbate these existing problems.

Psychological discomfort is another common cause of difficulty in either going to sleep or staying asleep. It is easy for a person's mind to become busy at night as the body relaxes and there are fewer distractions. Dwelling on problems or becoming anxious can prevent sleep long into the night.

If a person has disturbed nights, he may compensate for his lack of sleep by taking an afternoon nap. While this works for some people, it can further disrupt the usual routine, making the person more wakeful at night.

There are a number of practical steps you can take to help ensure a good night's sleep (see panel, below).

Disorders and sleep problems

There are some specific medical conditions that can cause difficulty with sleep.

■ **Dementia** This can further disrupt the normal daily cycle of activity and sleep. People with dementia may become very unsettled in the evening and sometimes throughout the night. Developing a night-time routine can be helpful: having the same drink and perhaps a snack, watching the television to settle, and using the same verbal prompts. If the person tends to wander at night, make sure the environment is safe and that the person cannot wander outside. A telecare or home call system (p.15) may help to keep a person who wanders safe at night by alerting you as his carer.

■ **Sleep apnoea** Someone with this disorder stops breathing repeatedly during sleep, leading to disturbed sleep. If the person is overweight, losing weight may help. Some people need to wear a mask at night that blows air or oxygen into the nose.

■ **Night-time hallucinations** These can be a feature of dementia and an effect of some medications, such as those for Parkinson's disease. In such cases a doctor may advise trying or changing medication to help.

TIPS FOR SLEEPING WELL

Here are a few suggestions that might help with sleep:

■ Make the bedroom a relaxing, peaceful place, with adequate warmth and fresh air.

■ Make sure the bed is comfortable.

■ Try to create a sleeping pattern, getting the person ready and into bed at a similar time each night, as well as up at a similar time.

■ Reading a book or watching gentle television can help a person relax, but avoid computer use or watching a high-speed, exciting television programme.

■ Maintain a healthy diet, but avoid eating a big meal late into the evening.

■ Cut down the amount of tea, coffee, alcohol, and fizzy drinks that are taken, and maybe reduce the amount of fluid that is drunk before bedtime. If the person wants an evening drink, try herbal tea or warm milk.

■ If the person is using regular pain medication, make sure this is taken in time so that it is working by the time he goes to bed.

■ Encourage the person to be as active as possible during the day, but not too close to bedtime.

■ If the person is a worrier, encourage him to learn relaxation techniques, and try to help him deal with his worries during the day, so that he can put them aside at night time.

BEDS AND BEDDING

Most people will continue to use their own bed while they are able to get in and out of it, or until they need care while in bed. If a bed is difficult to get in or out of because it is too low, it can be raised up on blocks (p.39). This also makes it easier for the carer to look after the person. There are also various devices that can make it easier for someone to turn over or sit up in bed (pp.39, 113, and 114).

Positioning of the bed

Wherever the bed is positioned within the room, it needs to be secure. If the person you are caring for is quite heavy, the bed may need to be braced against the wall, allowing him to push up from the bed, or sit down onto it, without risk of the bed moving.

If you, or another person, are caring for someone in bed, it needs to be away from the wall, allowing you access on both sides of the bed. See p.38 for how the bedroom might be arranged and suggestions for useful items to have handy near the bed.

Choosing bedding

Where possible, choose natural fibres for the bedding, such as cotton or cotton-mix sheets. Natural fibres breathe more easily, helping to regulate body heat. When caring for someone, duvets are generally easier to manage than sheets and blankets. Select a duvet that can be washed easily.

If the person you are caring for gets very sweaty at nights, you might consider moisture-wicking bedding and nightwear. These aim to draw any moisture away from the body and dry quickly.

If the person has a night-time incontinence, consider buying mattress and pillow protectors; there are also either washable or disposable absorbent pads available that fit across the bed under the person (p.138).

Changing the sheets

When you need to change the sheets, encourage the person you are caring for to get out of bed. However, ifshe is not able to do so, follow the method shown opposite.

SPECIAL BEDS

In the UK, electric adjustable beds, of the type used in hospitals, are sometimes provided for use at home. These are different from commercially available adjustable beds, which have a limited range of movement.

- Also called profiling beds, hospital beds have a head section that can be raised up; foot sections that can be angled into many positions (thus changing the bed's "profile"); and lockable wheels. The height of the bed can also be varied.

- The criteria for receiving a hospital bed may differ according to where a person lives.

- A person who needs nursing or personal care while lying on a bed, or who is unable to get on or off the bed without help and needs the additional variable height of a hospital bed, may meet the criteria.

- District nursing or occupational therapy services should be able to advise you.

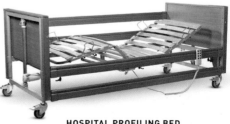

HOSPITAL PROFILING BED

People confined to bed are at risk of pressure sores (p.102). It is therefore very important that you smooth away any wrinkles in the bottom sheet so that they don't rub the skin. If using a top sheet, rather than a duvet, tuck it in loosely to allow free movement of the feet.

HOW TO CHANGE THE SHEETS OF A BEDBOUND PERSON

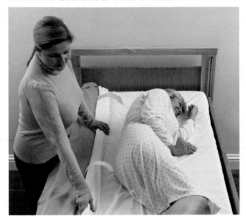

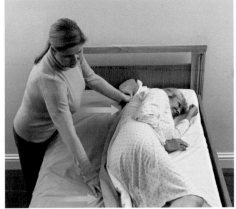

1 Have everything you need to hand. Remove the pillows and duvet, or top sheet and blankets. Ask the person to roll onto her side, assisting her if necessary (p.113). If you need to, take this opportunity to clean the person. Untuck the sheet on the near side of the bed. Roll it lengthways up to the person's back, catching any soiled material inside it.

2 Arrange the clean sheet on the near side of the bed, tucking the farther side under the roll of the soiled sheet if possible. Take care not to get the clean sheet dirty as you do so. Ask or assist the person to roll back towards you onto the clean sheet.

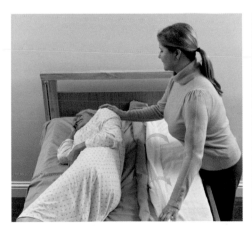

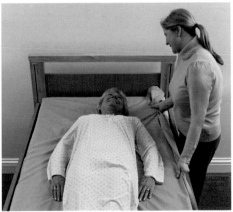

3 Once the person is in a comfortable, stable position on her side, walk round to the far side of the bed. Remove the soiled sheet. If you need to, take this opportunity to clean the person further.

4 Spread out the clean sheet on the far side of the person. Ask her to roll onto her back. You can now adjust the clean sheet as necessary. Finally, replace the pillows and bedclothes, making the person comfortable.

109

EQUIPMENT TO AID COMFORT

Whether a person is lying down to sleep or sitting up, perhaps to read or eat, it is important for him to be comfortable. Apart from bedding (p.108), there are a number of comfort aids that you might want to consider. Not only can they help him to sleep better and to enjoy activities in bed, but some also help to prevent pressure sores (p.102). Ask an occupational therapist for advice.

Support in bed

Good support is important if someone wants to sit up in bed. You can just provide plenty of ordinary pillows, placing them under the head, neck, shoulders, and arms for support. Alternatively, you might consider purchasing a special inverted-V-shaped pillow for support. Back rests and bed wedges are also available, against

Sitting up comfortably
An adjustable back rest allows a person to sit up in bed at whatever angle is most comfortable. It can be folded away when not in use.

Bed wedge
Made of foam, this is placed on top of the mattress against the bedboard to provide support for a person's back. Normal pillows can be placed on top of it for extra support.

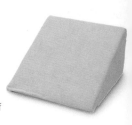

Bed roll
This can be placed under a person's knees to stop him sliding down the bed. It's useful when someone sleeps in a more upright position.

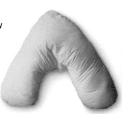

Inverted-V-shaped pillow
This pillow is shaped to provide even support for the head, neck, shoulders, and arms and enables a person to sit up comfortably.

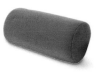

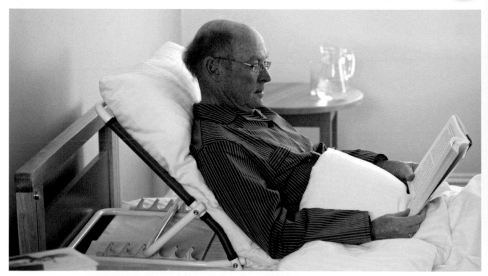

which pillows can be arranged. These supports can also be used if someone prefers to sleep in quite an upright position or has been advised to do so because of breathing difficulties.

Sometimes, when a person sleeps in a more upright position he tends to slip down the bed. This can be prevented by placing a pillow, a wedge, or a bed roll under the back of the knees.

Relieving pressure

People who spend long periods in bed are at risk of pressure sores. Special mattresses are available that help distribute pressure more evenly and a bed cradle can take the weight of bedclothes off vulnerable areas.

■ **Memory foam mattresses** Memory foam responds to body heat and weight by moulding to the contours of the person's body. A memory foam mattress helps to provide equally distributed support, so relieving particular pressure points.

■ **Air mattresses** Air-filled mattresses can be static or alternating. Static mattresses maintain a constant but low-pressure surface under the person. Alternating or cyclical pressure systems work by constantly inflating and deflating small sections of the mattress, so changing and relieving the pressure.

■ **Bed cradle** This is useful for someone who has very sore or swollen legs.

Staying warm

As people age, their ability to regulate and adjust body heat tends to diminish. An older person can be a degree or two cooler than average, especially if he is less mobile. Body temperature also tends to drop in the very early morning for everyone.

If possible any bedroom radiators or heaters should be thermostatically controlled. This allows the room to be

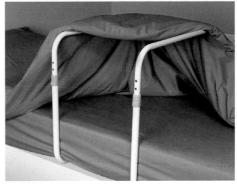

Bed cradle
This is a metal frame, the base of which slips between the mattress and the bed base. The top forms a support cradle for the bedclothes.

maintained at a steady temperature, rather than being too hot or cold.

Many people use hot-water bottles in bed. Those who do need to be aware of the risks of burns if a bottle that is too hot is placed directly on the skin, especially if the person has reduced sensation or is unable to move the bottle for himself. It is always advisable to use a bottle cover. There is also a risk if the person himself fills the bottle with very hot water but is unstable or has a tremor. There are alternative heat pads that you heat by microwaving for a short while.

Bed warmers are electrically heated mattress pads that are placed in the bed under the bottom sheet. They can be temperature controlled and have an inbuilt thermostat. They are not suitable for use on top of a pressure-relieving mattress as they reduce its effectiveness. Electric over-blankets are better in this circumstance. In both cases, manufacturers advise that they should not be used for people with reduced sensation. It is suggested they are not used by a person who is unable to manage the controls independently and safely.

In the UK, some councils offer an electric-blanket testing service to ensure that they are safe to use.

MOBILITY IN BED

Being mobile in bed and being able to get out of bed allows a person to participate in daily practical and social activities with less reliance on a carer. It is better for the person's circulation and breathing to be able to move about in the bed. With less mobility comes the risk of pressure sores (p.102) and stiffer, contracted joints.

If a person needs help changing position you can support him as he moves, but be careful you do not put stress on your own back, or pull on the person's joints. If the bed height is adjustable, raise the bed so that you do not have to bend.

Techniques for independent movement

Key abilities that enable independent movement in bed are bridging (below), shoulder or bottom walking (below, right), and rolling (opposite). These can be more difficult for a person to do if he is on an air or gel mattress, as the surface is less firm.

■ **Bridging** This position can be useful if you need to place a slide sheet under the person to move him up the bed, or for placing a bedpan under him.

■ **Bottom/shoulder walking** This is when the person "walks" his shoulders or bottom up or down the bed, by alternately lifting one side then the other off the mattress and shifting himself either up or down the bed. Bottom walking is also a good way for the person to move nearer the edge of the bed if he is sitting on the side, ready to stand up.

■ **Rolling** Rolling to one side is key to being able to get out of bed, or to adjusting position to avoid pressure sores. The person can hold onto a bed lever (a grab rail fitted onto the bed), or the bed sides to help him roll. If the person then wants to get out of bed, he can push up on his elbow or use the bed lever to pull himself up to sit on the edge of the bed (p.114).

Sitting up in bed

A person who wants to sit up in bed without getting out of bed may be able to do so with the help of a bed lever. A mattress elevator can also help: this is an electric frame that sits under the head end of the mattress. The person can use it (or it can be operated

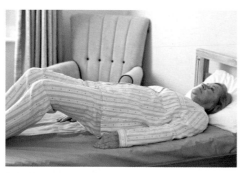

Bridging
The person lies on her back, with her hands by her sides. She draws her legs up to bend her knees, keeping her feet on the mattress. Using the back, tummy, and bottom muscles, she lifts her pelvis or bottom off the bed.

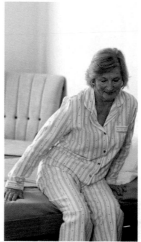

Bottom walking
The person lifts one side of her buttocks off the mattress, shifts it slightly forwards and replaces it on the mattress. She repeats this with the other side, and continues alternately lifting one side then the other.

WHEN NOT TO MOVE SOMEONE

In some situations, a person may benefit from remaining in bed if he is unwell or has a problem that is better dealt with in bed. Don't move the person if he:

- Is feeling dizzy or nauseous.
- Has had a fall leading to a possible injury.
- Is experiencing unusually severe joint pain.
- Has a pressure area or wound that would heal better in bed.

ROLLING INDEPENDENTLY

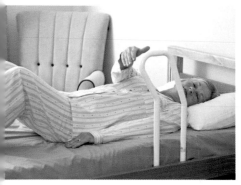

1 The person draws her legs up to bend her knees. She reaches one arm across her own body towards the side she is turning to, ready to grasp the bed lever (or bed side). She turns her head and shoulders towards the side.

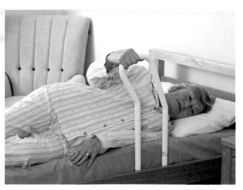

2 As she reaches across, gravity will help by tilting her bent knees towards the side. Holding onto the bed lever, or bed side, the person can pull herself over fully onto her side.

HELPING SOMEONE TO ROLL

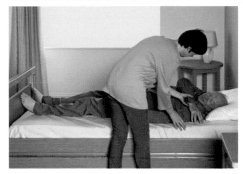

1 Place the arm nearest you slightly away from the person's body, so that it does not become trapped. Draw the farthest arm across his body, towards you. Do not pull on the limb, but support it as you lift.

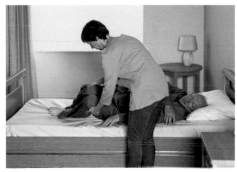

2 Help the person to bend his legs up. If he cannot manage to bend both legs, try to bend just the leg farthest from you.

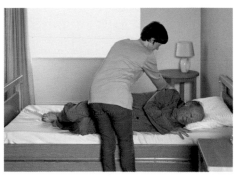

3 Put one hand on his farthest shoulder and one hand on his hip, and roll him towards you, onto his side.

» MOBILITY IN BED

GETTING OUT OF BED INDEPENDENTLY

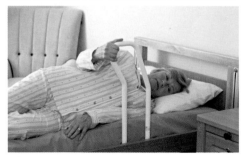

1 Encourage the person to roll onto her side towards you (p.113). She can then grasp the bed lever with her top hand.

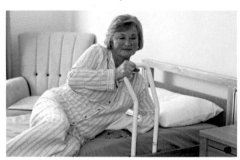

2 Ask her to slide her legs over the side of the bed As she does so, encourage her to push up on the bed with her elbow or pull on the bed lever to come up to a sitting position. Encourage her to move close enough to the edge of the bed so that her feet are flat on the floor. This might be by wriggling or by bottom walking (p.112).

SAFE HANDLING

When helping someone into a sitting position on the edge of the bed, there are some important safety considerations:

- Stand at the "top" end of the person to act as a barrier, which is opposite the chest and hip area (not at the head and not by the knees or feet).

- Once the person's feet are over the edge of the mattress he is vulnerable to falling out and should not be left in this position for long.

HELPING SOMEONE GET OUT OF BED

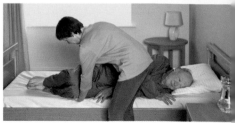

1 Help the person to roll onto his side (p.113). Place your hand under both knees and guide them towards the edge of the bed.

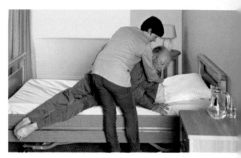

2 Support the person under his shoulder. Encourage him to use his upper hand to push up from the mattress, using the elbow of the other arm to support himself as he does so.

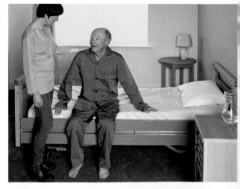

3 As his feet slide off the bed, the momentum helps him to swing up to a sitting position. Encourage him to wriggle or bottom walk (p.112) close enough to the edge of the bed so that his feet are flat on the floor.

by the carer) to sit up in bed, or lie down. Some designs have grab handles on the sides. A profiling bed (p.108), which has adjustable head and foot ends, can also help a person to sit up. Some people, however may require your help to sit up.

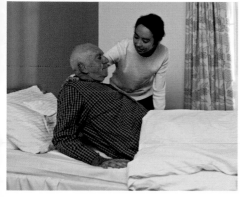

Helping someone to sit up
Place an arm around the person's shoulders and help him forwards.

Using a slide sheet to move someone

A slide sheet is a section of low-friction fabric that is used to move a person without the need for lifting, reducing any shearing forces on the person's skin. Slide sheets either come in pairs or are manufactured as a loop, creating two layers. They come in different sizes according to their use. Most assisted movements done with a slide sheet require two people to help.

USING A SLIDE SHEET TO MOVE SOMEONE UP THE BED

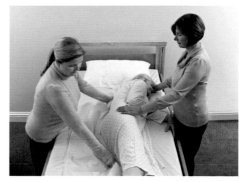

1 Help the person to roll to one side (p.113), then place the slide sheet behind her back, slightly tucked under her. You can also place a slide sheet by asking her to bridge (p.112).

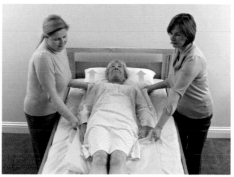

2 Roll her onto her back on top of the slide sheet. The slide sheet can be pulled through further, if necessary, so it can be reached on both sides. The carers grasp the top layer of the sheet and pull it towards the bed end.

POSITIONING IN BED AFTER SURGERY OR ILLNESS

Particular care must be taken with a person's position in bed after illness or surgery, so that affected limbs are supported and good posture and alignment are maintained.

Independent mobility in bed helps a person to stay in the correct position, which:

- Helps prevent possible contractures (shortening of muscles and tendons, which can lead to joint deformity).

- Maximizes muscle strength and joint flexibility.

- Minimizes and/or prevents pain.

- Prevents the development of pressure sores.

If the person has had a stroke (p.101), you may need to move his limbs for him. Limbs can be very heavy, so be aware of how you lift, protecting your back as you do so.

7

PERSONAL CARE

■ HELP WITH WASHING ■ HAIR CARE ■ CARE OF APPEARANCE
■ HAND AND FOOT CARE ■ MOUTH AND TOOTH CARE
■ CLOTHES AND DRESSING ■ USING THE TOILET
■ DEALING WITH INCONTINENCE
■ URINARY CATHETER CARE ■ STOMA CARE

HELP WITH WASHING

Good personal hygiene not only helps to prevent infection, but also keeps the skin in good condition and makes the person feel better about herself. As a carer, your role can vary from just helping with the preparation and being in the house in case of emergency, to physically assisting with washing and drying. Because of the intimate nature of personal hygiene, you should ask the person whether she would prefer assistance from a family member or someone else, such as a care assistant. Also ask whether she would prefer to have help from somebody of the same sex, although this may not always be possible.

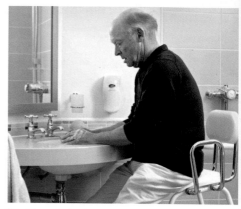

Washing at a basin
Using a chair or stool when washing at a basin can be helpful if a person has mobility problems or difficulty in standing for long periods.

Washing routines

Many people have set times and routines for washing and taking baths or showers, and preferences for, say, using a facecloth rather than a sponge and using talcum powder or not. You should try to maintain the person's routines and accommodate her preferences as much as possible. Once you have established a routine that suits both of you, try to stick to it. The person may not want a full shower or bath every day. If so, a simple wash at a basin is sufficient if there are no incontinence or medical issues that necessitate more thorough washing.

Showers and baths

There are several types of shower that can be used in the home, varying from using a shower-head attachment on the taps to wet rooms with full disability equipment installed. In general, shower units are

---

WASHING GUIDELINES

Follow the guidelines below to help ensure the person's safety and comfort while washing:

- Make sure the room is warm and well lit and that curtains (or blinds) and doors are closed.

- Check that there are no obstacles leading to, or in, the washing area.

- Make sure all equipment (e.g. shower seat, facecloth, and soap) is ready beforehand.

- Suggest that the person goes to the toilet before washing.

- Check the water temperature. Water in a shower must not be hotter than 41°C (106°F); water in a bath must not exceed 44°C (111°F).

- Let the person do as much as she can herself.

- If necessary, help with getting to the washing area and removing clothing.

- If the person needs help washing, wash from the face downwards to the feet. Wash all parts of the body, including under the breasts and arms, and the genital and anal areas.

- Help the person out of the washing area and dry her thoroughly.

more accessible than baths and so are easier to use for people with mobility problems. However, there are various ways in which a bath can be adapted to make it more accessible (p.40). If the person has difficulty turning on taps, try fitting adjustable tap turners or replace the taps with lever-style ones.

Helping someone to bathe

When helping somebody to bathe, you should let the person do as much herself as she can, both to help maintain her feeling of independence and to minimize strain on yourself. However, you must always check yourself that the water is at the correct temperature; bath temperature indicators (p.121) are useful for this.

You may wish to wear an apron to help keep you dry. When helping the person, it is also important to watch your position, to avoid getting back pain when leaning over or sore knees when kneeling. You may find it helpful to use long-handled sponges (p.121) or to sit on a small stool or chair. Kneel on rolled-up towels or cushions and alternate between sitting and standing.

When helping to dry the person, pat the skin rather than rubbing it, to avoid the possibility of damaging fragile skin. Several towels may be needed, one for modesty and others for drying. A towelling robe can be useful, helping to keep the person warm while drying at the same time.

Ensuring dignity and privacy

Washing is a very intimate act, and it is important to maintain the person's dignity. You want the experience to be as stress-free as possible for both of you. Having help with cleaning and personal hygiene can be embarrassing, especially if a member of the family is assisting. As the carer, you should try to act casually and relaxed, even if you don't feel that way. Imagine yourself in the person's place, and try not to show

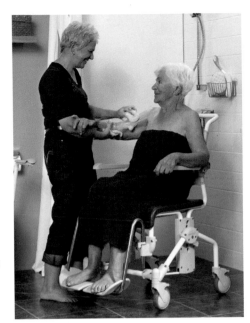

Helping a person wash
When helping someone to wash, keep her covered as much as practical to help maintain her dignity and minimize embarrassment.

that you are offended or embarrassed about anything. If you act in a calm way, then the person will also be calm. Be careful not to put yourself in any compromising position or act in any way that may provoke an inappropriate sexual reaction.

When helping with washing, always close the doors and curtains or blinds, even if nobody else is in the house. If you need to

SOAP OPTIONS

Various alternatives to ordinary soap are available, including:

- Clinical cleansing foam, which lathers more than ordinary soap and is more effective in cleaning.
- No-rinse soap or wipes, which just need to be rubbed in then towelled off. These save time and reduce the risk of soaking the bed when giving a bed bath.

›› HELP WITH WASHING

push the person through to the bathroom in a wheelchair or wheeled shower chair, cover her front and ensure that her bottom is not exposed.

When helping the person to dress, keep her lower body covered with a towel and dress her upper body first. The upper clothes then provide some modesty while dressing the lower part of her body.

The reluctant washer

If the person is reluctant or forgetful about washing, try to avoid confrontation and think about the washing routine the person used to have. Keep calm and allow time to discuss the situation and persuade the person. If her clothes need cleaning, that is a good opportunity to suggest that she undresses and has a wash before changing into clean clothes. Make sure the bathroom is warm before washing so that the person doesn't avoid undressing.

Giving a bed bath

If the person cannot get out of bed to wash, you will have to give a bedbath.

When giving a bedbath, the key thing is to be organized and gather all the necessary items beforehand. Ensure that there are plenty of towels and washcloths, and two bowls of water, one for washing and one for rinsing. A waterproof sheet or towels for placing under the person will prevent the mattress from getting soaked. You will also find it useful to have a table or trolley near at hand to place items on. Once you have all the items ready, make sure the room is warm and private.

GIVING A BED BATH

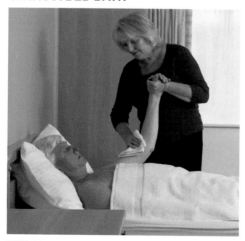

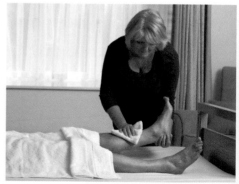

2 Finish washing one side of the body at the feet, then wash the other side, again starting at the head and working downwards. To clean the person's back, tilt him onto his side, then wash from the head downwards.

1 Undress the person but keep him covered with a blanket or large towel at all times, both to keep him warm and also to preserve his dignity. Start from the top of the body and work down one side. Only lift the cover away when you need to, and then replace it as soon as you have finished. Always rinse the soap off immediately, then pat the area dry.

3 It is generally easier and more hygienic to wash the genitals and anus last. The person will need to roll onto his side so that you can reach the rear, or it may be possible to reach from the front if he bends his knees. Be careful not to wipe any faecal material forwards.

LOOKING AFTER YOURSELF

Giving a bed bath can be physically demanding. There is also the possibility of hurting your back. Follow the guidelines below to minimize the physical stress and risk of back pain:

- The bed should be high enough that you don't risk hurting your back by having to bend over too much. If the person has an adjustable bed, raise or lower it to a suitable height. If the bed is not adjustable and is too low, it may be possible to raise it by placing blocks underneath (p.39). If a non-adjustable bed is too high, try standing on a stool.

- Don't be afraid to place your knee on the bed to lean over the person.

- Ask the person to give as much assistance as she can, for example by raising her arms or legs when necessary.

- Get assistance if you need help turning the person safely; extra help may be necessary even if all the correct disability equipment is in place.

- If you find giving bed baths too physically demanding, ask for help from your local authority or a local carers' organization.

EQUIPMENT FOR BATHING

EQUIPMENT	DESCRIPTION
Bath temperature indicators	■ Used to reduce the risk of scalding. ■ Some models fit in the plughole; others float in the water. ■ Can be preset to a safe temperature range.
Bath and shower mats	■ Used to prevent slipping. ■ Available in various shapes and sizes to fit different baths and shower units. ■ Choose a model that does not curl up at the edges and that has non-slip surfaces on the top and bottom.
Long-handled washing aids	■ Useful for people with restricted arm movement. ■ Available in different lengths and with different attachments, such as brushes and sponges. ■ Some models have pre-bent stems; others have flexible stems that can be bent to any shape required.
Double-sided flannel back strap	■ Useful for cleaning the back and the soles of the feet. ■ Consists of a long strap with soft terry cotton on one side and coarser foam on the other, and with an easy-to-grip handle at each end.
Toe washer	■ Useful for people who have difficulty bending down. ■ Consists of a long plastic handle that can be fitted with removable washing pads.

121

HAIR CARE

Having clean, well-groomed hair is an important part of personal hygiene and can also help to maintain a person's self-esteem and engender a positive outlook. As a carer, you should try to let the person look after her own hair as much as possible as this will help to maintain her sense of independence. You can help in this regard by providing special items that make basic hair care easier, such as long-handled brushes and combs. This section also provides advice on giving practical assistance, for example, in hair washing.

General care

Simply keeping the hair neat and tidy can be difficult, especially if a person has restricted shoulder or arm movement. Long-handled brushes and combs can help the person carry out basic hair care herself. Clippers can be useful for trimming hair, beards, and moustaches, and many come with special attachments for these purposes. Most clippers are rechargeable or battery-powered and are easy to use, either by you or the person in your care. If you are using heated rollers or tongs to style the person's hair, take care to avoid damaging the hair, especially if the person is elderly and has thin hair.

Long-handled brushes and combs
Some long-handled brushes and combs have large grip sections and are specially shaped to make it easier to reach the back of the head.

Going to the hairdresser

Going to the hairdresser or barber can be something to look forward to – a chance for the person to get out of the house and meet other people. However, it can be problematic, especially if the person has mobility problems. Try to find a hairdresser or barber that is on street level, has easy access, and can offer an alternative to washing the hair by leaning back over a basin. It may be better to have a dry cut or just a water spray to dampen the hair instead. Speak to the hairdresser or barber to see what they can offer. If going out to a hairdresser or barber is impractical, look for one that offers home visits.

Washing hair

The most convenient way to wash the person's hair is when she is having a bath or shower. There are special hair-washing trays that can be used over a basin, but they are primarily designed for people who are sitting in a chair or a wheelchair. The person must also be able to tip her head backwards to use the tray.

If the person wants to dry her own hair, she may find it easier by using a stand to support the hairdryer. Such stands are available from some specialist retailers.

Washing hair in bed

The easiest way to wash a person's hair while she is in bed is by using an inflatable wash basin. The basin is inflated and placed under the person's head, either on a low pillow or directly on the mattress. There is a tube at the side of the basin to allow water to drain out. When using an inflatable basin, place a waterproof cover or towel under it to protect the pillow and a bucket under the drainage tube to collect the waste water.

A plastic hair-washing tray can be used instead of an inflatable basin. These trays are similar to inflatable basins but do not hold as much water and have a drainage lip or spout rather than a tube. Trays also take up more storage space than inflatable basins and may be more uncomfortable. A portable shower bag can be a useful alternative to a jug for rinsing a person's hair in bed. These bags can hold up to about 10 litres (2.2 gal) of water and are

Using a hairdryer stand
Placing the hairdryer in a special stand makes hands-free drying possible. Some stands have a flexible neck so that the angle can be adjusted.

hung on a rail or hook above the bed head. The water flow is controlled with an on/off switch.

Wigs

Hair loss can be embarrassing and even frightening, especially for women. There are many reasons for hair loss, but if it is due to chemotherapy or certain skin diseases, then it is likely that, in the UK, a wig will be provided by the NHS. However, the person may have to pay for part or all of the cost, depending on her eligibility for help with the charges; the NHS website provides further information about this.

Alternatively, wigs can be bought privately.

A wig may be completely artificial or may be made of various proportions of human hair. It is important for the person to consider whether she wants to wear a wig or would prefer to wear nothing or possibly a scarf or bandana instead. If the person does opt for a wig, she will need to get it specially fitted.

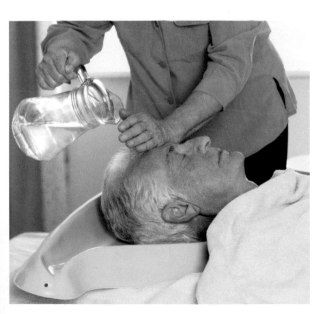

Using a hair-washing tray
The tray is placed under the person's head and collects waste water, which drains out through a lip or spout into a bucket placed on the floor.

CARE OF APPEARANCE

Most people have a particular perception of themselves and how they like to appear to others. Some take extreme pride and care in appearing well-groomed, whereas others may prefer a more natural look. A person's appearance can help define her role and identity – it is part of who she is. If it is difficult to maintain this appearance, perhaps due to frailty or physical or mental limitations, this can have a significant effect on psychological wellbeing.

As a carer, you should be alert to signs that the person is having problems in looking after her appearance. Such signs are often easy to spot – for example, the person may no longer be able to apply make-up properly or may find it difficult to put on jewellery. If you notice such signs, you should try to find out the underlying cause. It could be something simple like a poor grip or shaky hands, or the person may be depressed and/or confused. Finding a solution may involve getting a piece of equipment to make a specific task easier, assisting the person, or seeking professional help if you suspect a medical problem.

TIPS FOR MAKE-UP

If applying or choosing appropriate make-up is problematic, the tips below may prove useful:

- Tweezers with a magnifier attachment may be helpful for those who have reduced sight but a steady hand.

- Long-handled sponge applicators make it easier to apply lotion or moisturizer to the lower legs or back.

- Tinted moisturizer a shade lighter than the person's actual skin tone can help to soften the appearance of wrinkles. It is also less likely than a concealer to stick in creases.

- Let the person choose the make-up she wants to put on, then remove all other products. This avoids the temptation of applying too much make-up.

- Try to arrange a home visit from a cosmetics company or promoter to advise on suitable products.

Applying make-up

If a person has always worn make-up, she may not feel normal without it and may also have strong preferences about the type and style of make-up and how it is applied. You should try to accommodate such preferences, if possible, although they may need to be adapted. For example, some make-up requires a lot of dexterity to apply, such as mascara. If the person is not able to apply mascara properly, not only could the final result

Applying make-up
When applying make-up, allow the person herself to choose the product and follow her preferences about how she would like the product applied.

look unattractive but there is also the potential risk of damage to the eyes. In this situation, you should try to persuade her to let you apply the mascara or you could even suggest that she stops using it completely.

If the person has a weak grip, you can try padding the handles of make-up applicators with foam tubing to make them easier to hold. Also consider buying special brushes or sponges with wide, easy-to-grip handles.

If the person has poor eyesight, she may not be able to see well enough to apply make-up properly or even differentiate between its colours, and the final effect may be overdone. It may be possible to compensate for poor vision by good lighting and using a magnifier, such as a magnifying mirror. If the person normally wears glasses for near vision, encourage her to use them when applying lipstick.

Shaving

Electric shavers are generally easier to use than traditional razors and also minimize the risk of cuts and abrasions. Most electric shavers have large handles or grip sections, which make them easy to hold. Shaving with an electric shaver is also quicker and less messy than a wet shave with a traditional razor. However, if the person does prefer a wet shave but is unable to shave himself safely – perhaps because of poor eyesight, a weak grip, or a tremor – then you should shave him yourself. In such cases, it may be advisable to try to convert the person to using an electric razor. This can be done

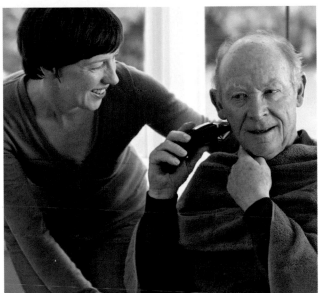

Using an electric shaver
An electric shaver may enable a person to continue to shave himself when it would not be safe to do so using a traditional razor.

gradually, for example by alternating between using an electric shaver and giving wet shaves, then slowly reducing the frequency of wet shaves.

If the person shaves himself, he may find a weighted holder helps to keep the razor or shaver steady. A razor or shaver can also be adapted to make it easier to hold by attaching a cuff that wraps around the hand. These cuffs can be bought from specialist retailers, or you can make your own by gluing a strip of elastic or Velcro to the handle of the razor or shaver.

Whether you shave the person or he shaves himself, the area should be well lit. It is also advisable that he is sitting down during the process. A mirror (preferably a shaving mirror that produces a magnified reflection) is essential if the person is shaving himself, but it is also useful if you are shaving him as it will enable him to see what you are doing.

HAND AND FOOT CARE

Proper hand and foot care is often overlooked but it is just as important as other aspects of personal care. The hands and feet should be cleaned and moisturized regularly, and the nails should be kept trimmed. If you have concerns about foot and nail care, it may be beneficial to contact a local chiropodist. Some offer a nail-cutting service and may also carry out home visits.

Cutting nails

Nails generally harden with age and it is easier to cut them after a shower or bath. For cutting fingernails, nail clippers with an attached magnifier are useful for those who have poor eyesight. It is also possible to buy nail clippers with a suction pad that can be attached to a flat surface and used one-handed. Suction nail brushes are also available.

If it is difficult for the person to reach down to cut her toenails, she could try using long-handled nail scissors. However, because of the risk of accidental injury, these should only be used if the person has good eyesight and manual dexterity. Otherwise, you should cut the person's toenails yourself or get a chiropodist to

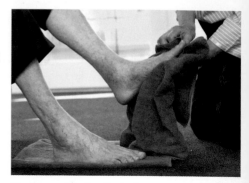

Washing and drying the feet
The feet should be washed and dried thoroughly, especially between the toes, to reduce the risk of a fungal infection such as athlete's foot.

do so. Toenails should always be cut straight across, to avoid ingrowing toenails. Nail clippers are often better than scissors for this.

Looking after the feet

Foot care is essential for everybody, but it is especially important if the person has a disorder such as diabetes or a circulation problem, in order to prevent potentially serious complications from developing.

As a carer, you should check the person's feet every week, and, if you notice any problems, deal with them at once (see table, opposite). The feet should be washed and dried thoroughly (particularly between the toes) every day. If the person washes her own feet, long-handled toe washers (p.121) can be useful. Applying moisturizer after washing will help to prevent dry skin. Footwear should fit properly, without pinching or squashing the toes, and socks should be changed daily. In bed, gel or wheat warmers are preferable to hot-water bottles. If an electric blanket is used, you should make sure it is turned off before the person goes to bed.

BRITTLE NAILS

Brittle nails are usually just due to aging or overexposure to water or chemicals such as detergents, although sometimes they may be a sign of an underlying disorder. If brittle nails are a problem, try the following:

- Make sure gloves are worn for wet tasks, such as washing up.

- Apply moisturizing cream frequently.

- Try using a nail hardener.

- If the above measures don't work or there are additional symptoms, consult a doctor.

COMMON FOOT PROBLEMS

PROBLEM	POSSIBLE CAUSE	ACTION
Corns and calluses (localized areas of hard, thickened skin)	Pressure, often from poorly fitting footwear	■ Soak the feet to soften the skin and rub the corn or callus with a pumice stone to remove the thickened skin. If the person has diabetes, consult a doctor before removing thickened skin. ■ Apply adhesive sponge padding over the affected area. ■ Ensure the person wears well-fitting footwear. ■ If the above measures do not help, consult a chiropodist.
Bunion (thickened tissue over the joint at the base of the big toe)	Misaligned joint at the base of the big toe	■ Ensure the person wears well-fitting footwear to reduce pressure on the joint. ■ If a bunion is painful or a cause for concern, consult a doctor.
Sore, peeling, itchy skin between the toes	Athlete's foot (a fungal infection)	■ Wash and dry the feet and apply an over-the-counter antifungal preparation. ■ If symptoms last for more than two weeks, consult a doctor. ■ If redness and swelling develop, consult a doctor at once.
Cracked heels	Accumulation of hard, dry skin on the heels	■ Soak the feet to soften the skin and remove hard skin with a pumice stone. Apply a moisturizer. If the person has diabetes, consult a doctor before removing the hard skin.
Redness and swelling around the edge of a toenail	Ingrowing toenail	■ Wash the feet regularly using soap and water. ■ Gently push the skin away from the ingrowing nail using a cotton bud. ■ Ensure the person wears footwear with plenty of space around the toes. ■ If the toenail is painful, give paracetamol; to avoid a possible overdose, first check that the person has not taken other medications that contain paracetamol. ■ If the toenail does not improve or other symptoms develop, consult a doctor.
Painful, pale or blue-tinged feet	Circulation problem	■ Consult a doctor at once.
Painful toe joints	Arthritis or gout	■ Consult a doctor.

MOUTH AND TOOTH CARE

Maintaining good oral hygiene helps to prevent tooth decay, mouth infections, and bad breath. It is especially important if the person is elderly because, as we age, less saliva (which helps to keep teeth clean) is produced and the gums recede. Signs that a person is having difficulty with mouth and tooth care include bad breath, stained teeth, food debris on the teeth, and red gums. As a carer, you should check that the person is managing to maintain good oral hygiene – or provide help if necessary – and also has regular dental checkups.

Routine care

Teeth should be brushed twice a day with a fluoride toothpaste for at least two minutes. The best times are first thing in the morning and last thing at night. The teeth should not be brushed immediately after a meal because this can damage the teeth. A manual or electric toothbrush can be used, but electric ones are more efficient at cleaning and are also easier to hold because of their larger handles.

When brushing, the teeth should be brushed on all sides. If a manual toothbrush is used, the teeth should be brushed with small, circular movements. The tongue should also be brushed lightly to reduce the build-up of "fur".

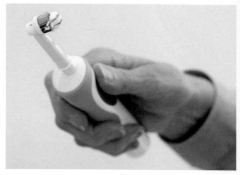

Using an electric toothbrush
Electric toothbrushes are easier to use than manual brushes, because they have large handles and require less effort when brushing.

The teeth should also be flossed every day. If normal floss is too difficult to manage, special floss holders with wide handles and electric flossers are available.

After brushing and flossing, the mouth should be rinsed. If a mouthwash is used, avoid ones that contain alcohol, as they can dry out the mouth and lips.

■ **Dentures** These should be cleaned as often as normal teeth. They should be removed, brushed with toothpaste, then soaked in a special denture-cleaning solution. After soaking, they should be brushed again before being put back in the mouth. It is also important that they are checked regularly by a dentist for fit, because poorly fitting dentures can cause discomfort and may also lead to sores, mouth infections, or problems with eating and speaking.

Help with tooth care

Two of the more common reasons why a person may need help with tooth care are poor hand control and dementia.

■ **Poor hand control** If the person has a weak grip or poor hand control, simply

---

TIPS FOR GOOD ORAL HYGIENE

Follow the recommendations below to help keep the mouth and teeth healthy:

- ■ Brush the teeth twice a day and floss once a day.
- ■ Don't smoke – smoking stains the teeth, causes bad breath, damages the gums, and may lead to oral cancer.
- ■ Eat a healthy diet.

COMMON MOUTH PROBLEMS

PROBLEM	POSSIBLE CAUSE	ACTION
Dry mouth	A dry mouth may be a side effect of some medications or a symptom of certain diseases, such as Sjogren's syndrome (an immune system disorder).	■ The person should avoid alcohol and should not smoke. ■ Give the person sugar-free sweets or gum to stimulate salivation. ■ Consult a doctor if the dry mouth persists or is accompanied by other symptoms.
Cold sores	Usually occurring around the lips, cold sores are caused by infection with the herpes simplex virus. After the virus is contracted, it becomes dormant but can then be reactivated later, resulting in an outbreak of cold sores. Factors that may trigger reactivation include stress, fever, trauma, hormonal changes, and exposure to sunlight. Cold sores are highly contagious until they have healed completely.	■ Ensure the person does not pick or squeeze the sores; hands should be washed after touching the sores. ■ The person should avoid close contact with others until the sores have healed. ■ Apply a cold sore cream as soon as the first signs appear (a tingling sensation around the mouth). ■ Consult a doctor if cold sores do not clear up within three weeks.
Canker sores (also called aphthous ulcers)	Typically found on the inside of the cheek or lip or under the tongue, canker sores can have many causes, including injury, immune deficiency, stress, allergy, and hormonal changes. They are not contagious.	■ Apply an analgesic mouth gel. ■ The person should use a soft toothbrush and eat soft foods to avoid irritating the sores. ■ Consult a doctor if the sores are very painful or do not heal by themselves.

holding a toothbrush, even a large electric one, may be difficult. It may help to make the handle of the brush larger by padding it with foam. Alternatively, try putting a Velcro strap around the handle of the brush and over the person's hand. It may also be possible to use a universal cuff or a large handle normally used for cutlery.

If the person finds it difficult to squeeze out toothpaste from a tube, toothpaste in a pump-action dispenser may be easier to use. There are also special toothpaste squeezers available. Some come with stands or wall brackets to enable one-handed operation.

■ **Dementia** If the person is confused or suffering from dementia, she is likely to neglect her teeth or may even forget how to brush properly. Sometimes, all that's necessary is a verbal prompt or giving the person the toothbrush with toothpaste already on it. Or a mime of how to brush may be enough to make the person understand what to do. However, you may have to help to complete the brushing and make sure it has been done thoroughly. You should also ensure that the person does not swallow mouthwash.

Toothpaste squeezer
There are many different types of toothpaste squeezers available. The one shown here can be used one-handed.

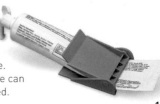

129

CLOTHES AND DRESSING

Most of us like to choose what we wear, and our clothing often reflects our personality or how we feel. Getting dressed is usually a private activity but, as a carer, you may just need to remind the person to dress and undress, or you may need to offer physical assistance. The key thing to remember when assisting the person is to respect her choices, privacy, and dignity.

Allowing time for dressing

Don't rush the person, and allow her plenty of time to dress. If you are in a hurry, the likelihood is that you will do everything for the person to speed up the process. However, over time, this de-skills the person and eventually she may no longer be able to dress without help, which will place more responsibility for caring on you. If you are in a rush on a particular day, a compromise is to have everything organized the night before. Then assist only with any specific tasks the person finds especially difficult – doing up buttons, for example.

Choosing clothes

Clothes are a very personal choice so it is important to involve the person herself as much as possible when buying them. Try to go shopping together or, if that isn't possible, look at catalogues or websites.

If you have to choose clothes, try to pick the type, style, and colours you know the person likes. However, you should also take into account any specfic problems the person may have, such as a weak grip, restricted joint movements, problems with fine finger control, or poor eyesight, as these may make some clothes more difficult to put on or take off. Similarly, if a person uses a wheelchair or is bedbound, then certain styles of clothing will be more suitable than others.

TIPS FOR CHOOSING SUITABLE CLOTHES

If a person has difficulty with dressing, the tips here may be helpful when choosing clothes:

- Choose clothing that is not too tight. It may be necessary to buy a size larger than normal as clothes with tight sleeves can restrict and are difficult to take off.

- Front-opening tops and dresses are generally easier for people who cannot raise their hands over their heads.

- For women, front- or side-opening skirts and trousers, or wraparound skirts, are easier than back-opening ones.

- Choose clothes with large buttons rather than poppers. If a favourite item has small buttons, it may be possible to put it over the head like a jumper and then only the top buttons will need fastening.

- Men may find it easier to put on boxer shorts rather than tight-fitting pants.

- Flannelette and cotton nightwear may stick to sheets and make turning over in bed difficult. Choose more "slippery" materials, but make sure they are breathable.

- Some companies make clothes that have back openings specifically for people who use a wheelchair.

- Many types of bra are difficult to put on independently. With a back-opening bra, try fastening it at the front then twisting it around. Otherwise, consider front-fastening or pull-over bras, or support vests. Some companies make bras with magnetic or Velcro fastenings that are easier to put on.

- Slip-on shoes and those with elastic laces or Velcro fastenings are easier to put on and take off. Slippers should only be worn for short periods because they do not provide adequate support for walking around safely indoors.

If the person likes a particular item of clothing and it is easy to put on, then it is sensible to suggest buying several, perhaps in different colours. If the person is happy to leave the choice up to you, stick to what you know works.

Washing and ironing clothes may be tasks that the person finds difficult, so look for easy-care fabrics that dry quickly and require little or no ironing.

When choosing which clothes to wear, layers of clothing are often a good idea, particularly if the person is elderly, because older people often feel the cold but can easily get overheated when the temperature rises.

■ **Making alterations** If the person finds her existing clothes difficult to put on, it may be possible to alter them rather than buying new clothes – for example by changing fastenings to Velcro or fitting loops to the end of zips. If you can't make such alterations yourself, you could try using a professional alteration service.

Assisting with dressing

When helping a person to dress, let her do as much as she can herself. You should also respect her choice of clothing, even if it looks strange to you. However, if the

> ### HELPING A PERSON WITH DEMENTIA
>
> If the person has dementia, limiting the amount of choice and organizing the clothing in an easy-to-understand and systematic way can often be helpful.
>
> ■ Keep items that are commonly used, such as underwear, in a drawer that is easy to find and access.
>
> ■ Put labels or pictures on drawers describing the contents.
>
> ■ Put items that are not used regularly at the back of a wardrobe or in another room.

clothes she chooses are completely unsuitable for the weather or may cause offence, you should tactfully point out the problem and guide her towards more appropriate clothing.

You should try to follow the person's normal dressing routine, although it may be sometimes be necessary to change it for safety. For example, if the person has problems with balance, she should dress sitting in a chair rather than on a bed. If the person is confused or has dementia, she may also need verbal prompting about the sequence of dressing, how to put on items of clothing, or how to use an aid such as a button hook.

HELPING SOMEONE TO DRESS

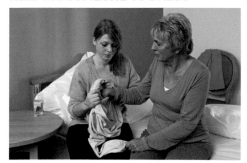

1 Make sure the person is sitting safely, either on a bed or, if the person has balance problems, on a chair. Help the person put her weaker limb in the item of clothing.

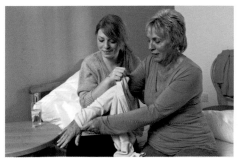

2 Help the person put on the rest of the garment, finishing with the stronger limb. When helping with undressing, start with the stronger limb and finish with the weaker one.

» CLOTHES AND DRESSING

Self-dressing aids

There are various items of equipment available that make it easier for a person to dress herself. These are generally divided into aids for dressing the upper half of the body and aids for the lower half. Practice is required with all such aids, and it is advisable to have a demonstration before purchase.

Common physical difficulties when dressing the upper half of the body are placing items over the head, doing up bras, and reaching around the back to pull and adjust garments. The main difficulty when dressing the lower half of the body is reaching down to the feet to put on socks and shoes or pull on items like pants or trousers. If the person has a weak grip, fastenings such as zips and buttons can can be a problem whether dressing the upper or lower half of the body. Some of the more useful aids are described below.

■ **Button hook and zip puller** Most button hooks consist of a shaped wire to place over the button and a large handle for easy grip. Some also have a hook on the end of the handle to pull zips. Separate zip pullers are also available. There are several different designs but many consist simply

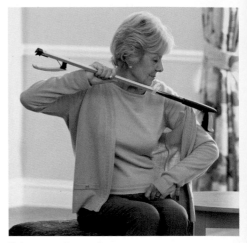

Using a reacher to dress
A reacher can be used instead of a dressing stick to help with dressing. The jaws can be used to grip part of a garment, and the trigger can be used as a hook, as shown here.

of an easy-grip handle with a long, large hook for putting through the hole of a zip puller tab.

■ **Dressing stick** This is a particularly useful piece of equipment if a person's shoulder movement is limited. Most dressing sticks have a similar design, consisting of a long, easy-grip handle with a large combination hook/pusher at one end. The large hook is used to lift a garment over the head. The pusher is used to push the garment off the shoulders. Some also have a small hook at the other end for pulling zips and shoelace loops. Although not designed specifically for dressing, a reacher can often be used instead of a dressing stick.

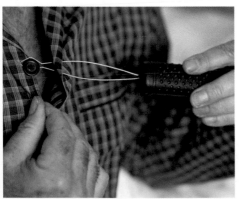

Using a button hook
Put the wire through the buttonhole and over the button, then pull on the handle with a twisting motion to draw the button through the buttonhole.

If the person finds it difficult to manage normal shoelaces, try the options below:

- Elastic laces can convert shoes into a slip-on style. When putting shoes on, take care that the tongue does not curl under; it may be necessary to thread the lace through the tongue to avoid this.
- Coiler laces are like springs. They thread through the eyelets like normal laces but are simply pulled to the desired tension and do not need tying.

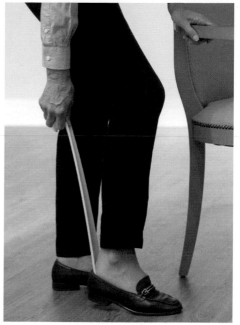

Using a long-handled shoehorn
Place the end of the shoehorn in the heel of the shoe, then ease the foot into the shoe while simultaneously pulling out the shoehorn.

- **Reacher** This device consists of a long handle with jaws at one end and a trigger for operating the jaws at the other. Reachers are available in different lengths and with different grips. Many have a magnet at one end for picking up metal objects, and some have locking jaws. Reachers are designed for picking up objects that are out of reach, but many people also find them useful for dressing.
- **Sock and tights aids** These come in a variety of styles. One of the most common types consists of a plastic "trough" with a ribbon at each end. Other types include ones with a flexible cloth-lined trough or a double trough for putting on tights.

- **Long-handled shoehorn** These are available in different lengths, and some also have a hook at the end, enabling them to be used as a reacher.

HOW TO USE A SOCK AID

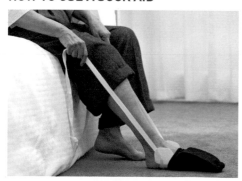

1 Put the trough into the sock, making sure the top of the sock is in the notches on either side of the trough, then grasp the ribbons and slowly pull.

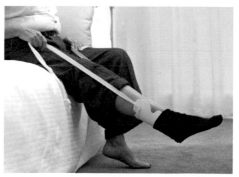

2 Keep pulling on the ribbons to draw the sock onto the foot. When the sock is all the way on, continue to pull on the ribbons to remove the trough.

USING THE TOILET

Going to the toilet is usually a private matter and it can be embarrassing for both the person and carer when assistance is necessary. There are many aids available that make it easier to use the toilet and these may enable the person to manage with minimal or even no help. However, if the person does require assistance, you should give her as much privacy as possible and always take care to preserve her dignity.

Accessing the toilet area
If there are concerns about the person's mobility or mental state, she may need supervision to get to the toilet. You may need to help her to stand up and walk, hold doors open, or even adjust clothes. As the carer, you will know the person's abilities, when she can manage by herself, and when she needs assistance.

Make sure there are no obstacles on the way to the toilet, for example by moving

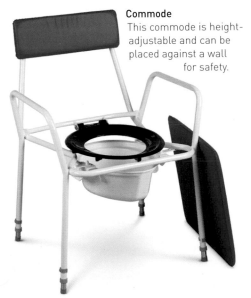

Commode
This commode is height-adjustable and can be placed against a wall for safety.

furniture to allow easier access for a walking frame or wheelchair, or removing loose rugs. Raised thresholds between doorways can be a hazard and these may need lowering. Make sure the route to the toilet is well lit, especially at night, and that lights can be switched on and off easily. Motion-sensor lights can be helpful. Alternatively, fit light switches with large on/off buttons or pull cords. Encourage the person to leave the door unlocked when using the toilet, in case of emergency, or fit a lock that can be opened from the outside.

To make using the toilet easier for a person with dementia and/or confusion, put a sign or a picture on the toilet door. Try to leave the door slightly ajar when the toilet is not in use, otherwise the person may think that the room is occupied.

If there is no access to a toilet on the same level as the living or sleeping area, it may be possible to fit a stair lift or even to adapt the home to add another toilet (see pp.28–41 for more advice). Other options include using a commode or chemical toilet.

Helping the person use the toilet
If the person is elderly or has dementia, she may need reminders to go to the toilet. In such cases, it's a good idea to have set times and a set routine, for example every two hours or before meals. The reminders can be verbal, gentle physical guidance, or even via a telecare service (p.15).

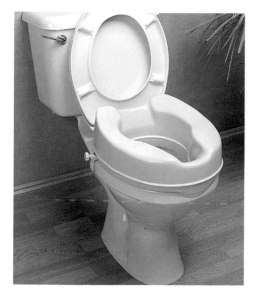

Raised toilet seat
Most raised toilet seats are designed to fit on normal toilets. Some models are available in different heights or are height-adjustable.

Toilet equipment
There is a wide variety of equipment available to help those with difficulty in using the toilet, including special toilet seats, support rails and toilet frames, and commodes. There are also urinals and, for those who are bedbound or wheelchair-dependent, bedpans.

■ **Toilet seats** Raised toilet seats are available for those who have difficulty in sitting down or standing up. There are many different models, but most are easy to fit to normal toilets. With some models, it is possible to adjust the height; some also have arms to further aid standing up and sitting down.

■ **Support rails and frames** Support rails are mounted on the wall or floor next to the toilet (pp.40–41). They must have a secure mounting as they must be able to bear the person's weight. An alternative option is a toilet frame. Most frames are free-standing

When going to the toilet, the person may need assistance with her clothing. She may also need help with wiping, although, if possible, she should be allowed to do this herself. It is important that wiping is done properly – from front to back – both for cleanliness and to reduce the risk of infection. Moist wipes may be better than ordinary toilet paper, as they are easier to hold and more effective at cleaning.

If there are mild problems of soiling, it may be because the person is not able to reach. In such cases, a long-handled bottom wiper may help. This acts like an extended arm, with a gripper to hold the paper on one end. Some also have a quick-release button on the other end, so that the soiled paper can be discarded without having to touch it. Bottom wipers should be cleaned thoroughly and disinfected after every use. It may be helpful to have several, so that a clean one is always immediately available. A bidet may also be useful; portable ones can be fitted to the toilet for temporary use. It is possible to get combined toilet and bidet units, some of which include warm-air dryers.

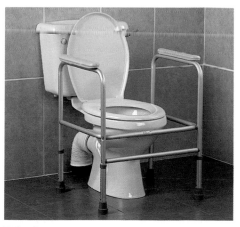

Toilet frame
Frames that fit around the toilet are useful for those who need support. Many are height-adjustable, and some are also width-adjustable.

» USING THE TOILET

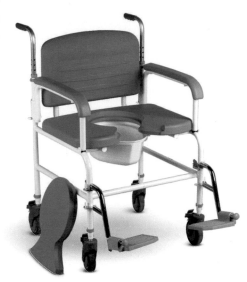

Mobile commode
A mobile commode is essentially a standard commode with wheels and brakes. Some have extra features, such as footrests, adjustable or removable arms, and a lid.

and can be adjusted for height. Some can also be adjusted for width, and certain models have accessories that enable them to be used as shower seats.

■ **Commodes** The standard commode is a chair with arms and a removable seat. Underneath there is a pan that can be removed easily for emptying. Commodes can be fixed height or adjustable, and some have removable arms for sideways access.

Care must be taken when using a commode because of the risk of it tilting backwards if the person sits down heavily. For this reason, it is safer to place a commode against a wall.

With certain models, it is possible to use them as a commode, or they can be placed over a toilet and used as a movable toilet frame. Other models are also suitable for use as shower chairs.

Folding commodes are also available for temporary use or when on holiday.

■ **Mobile commodes** These are similar to standard commodes but have wheels and brakes; some also have footrests and adjustable or removable arms.

■ **Urinals** Most people think of urinals as being suitable only for men, but there are also urinals for women and some that can be used by both sexes. The standard male urinal can be used when in bed, sitting, or standing. Most have a spill-proof lid and a holder to attach them to the side of a bed. The standard type of female urinal has an anatomically shaped opening and can be used when in bed, sitting, or standing, although most do not have a spill-proof lid. The female slipper urinal is designed primarily for those who are bedbound or use a wheelchair. Shaped like a bedpan, it has an end-cap for emptying.

It is also possible to get compact travel urinals (male, female, and unisex), which can be useful when away from home and with no access to a toilet.

■ **Bedpans** These can be used for urination and/or defecation while lying in bed. There are various designs, some with handles to aid positioning and a lid. Bedpan liners are also available to make disposal of the contents easier.

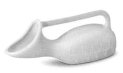

Urinal for women
Typically, a female urinal consists of a plastic container with an anatomically shaped opening.

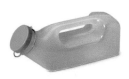

Urinal for men
Most male urinals consist of a plastic container with a retained lid to prevent spillage.

DEALING WITH INCONTINENCE

Incontinence can have a significant effect on a person's quality of life and can also be difficult for you as the carer. However, whether the person has urinary or faecal incontinence, or both, there are many practical things you can do to minimize its impact. You should also consult a doctor as there may be treatments that can help.

Urinary incontinence

There are several types of urinary incontinence, the most common being stress incontinence and urge incontinence. In stress incontinence, an activity such as coughing, sneezing, or physical exertion causes involuntary release of urine. In urge incontinence – also known as irritable bladder – there is an urgent desire to pass urine followed by involuntary urination. Total incontinence is complete lack of bladder control. It is comparatively uncommon and is often due to a nervous system disorder, such as a spinal cord injury or dementia.

Dealing with urinary incontinence

There are many ways in which incontinence can be managed so that it is less of a problem, both for you and the person you are caring for. It is generally best to start with methods to promote continence. Sometimes, these will be enough by themselves to deal with the problem effectively. In other cases, it may also be necessary to use incontinence aids.

■ **Promoting continence** It is often possible to minimize the problem of incontinence by altering the person's routines or behaviours.

Encourage the person to drink less in the evening before bed and to avoid drinks that stimulate urination, such as tea, coffee, and alcohol.

If the person has been prescribed diuretics, give the last dose well before bedtime to reduce the likelihood of the person having to get up in the night to urinate. However, you should consult a doctor before altering the person's drug regimen.

PELVIC FLOOR EXERCISES

The pelvic floor is a sheet of muscles between the legs, running from the pubic bone at the front to the base of the spine at the rear. The muscles support the abdominal organs and are also used to urinate. Exercising the muscles can help to strengthen them, which may help improve urinary incontinence, particularly stress incontinence, in men and women.

■ Pelvic floor exercises can be done sitting, standing, or lying down, but initially the person may find it easier to do them when sitting.

■ Get the person to identify her pelvic floor muscles: they are the ones that can be felt tightening when the flow of urine is stopped in midstream.

■ The person should then tighten the muscles and keep them tightened for 10 seconds, then relax; this should be repeated 10 times.

■ Alternatively, the person should tighten the muscles and hold them like this for as long as possible, then slowly relax; this should be repeated six times.

■ The person should not hold her breath or tighten her abdominal, buttock, or thigh muscles while performing the exercises.

■ Initially, the exercises should be done three to four times a day. When incontinence starts to improve, which may take several weeks, this can be reduced to twice a day.

■ The exercises should be continued even when incontinence improves; otherwise, the problem may return.

» DEALING WITH INCONTINENCE

Encourage the person to empty her bladder completely before going to bed. Sometimes it helps if the person goes to the toilet once then tries again a few minutes later.

Put a commode or urinal right next to the bed so that the person does not have to make a trip to the bathroom. Make sure there is a bedside light so that the person can see as she gets out of bed.

Encourage the person to perform pelvic floor exercises regularly (p.137). These can be done by men and women and are particularly useful for improving stress incontinence.

■ **Incontinence aids** There are a large number of products available to help with incontinence. If methods to promote continence are not completely effective, such aids can make a significant difference to the person's quality of life – for example,

by enabling her to go out with confidence. They can also make life easier and less stressful for you as the carer.

Incontinence pads and liners are available for both men and women in different sizes and with different degrees of absorbency. They wick moisture away from the body in much the same way as disposable nappies. Most pads and liners are worn with normal underwear, although there are also special incontinence pants. Usually, these products are discarded when soiled, but it is also possible to obtain washable pads, liners, and pants that can be reused. In general, pads and liners are suitable for mild incontinence, while pants are preferable for more severe incontinence. Some women may try using sanitary pads, but this is not recommended as they are not designed for incontinence and will remain damp.

PERSONAL INCONTINENCE AIDS

The most suitable type of incontinence aid will depend partly on the person's own preference and partly on the severity and type of incontinence. Some of the more common types are shown below.

■ **Female urinary incontinence pads** These are available with different degrees of absorbency and are usually shaped to fit inside either non-stretch or stretch underwear.

■ **Male urinary incontinence pads** These are similar to female pads but are anatomically shaped for men.

■ **Urinary incontinence pants** These usually have high absorbency for more severe urinary incontinence.

■ **Faecal incontinence pants** Nappy-style pants are generally more suitable for faecal incontinence. Many types can also be used for severe urinary incontinence.

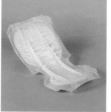

FEMALE URINARY INCONTINENCE PADS

MALE URINARY INCONTINENCE PAD

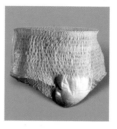

URINARY INCONTINENCE PANTS

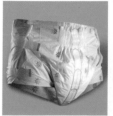

FAECAL INCONTINENCE PANTS

As well as personal incontinence aids, there are also various products to protect beds and chairs. They will also help to prevent the person from developing pressure sores (p.102) and skin infections.

Bed pads with a waterproof backing are available in different sizes. They may be disposable or washable, and some can be tucked in so that they don't move at night. A washable, waterproof mattress cover can also be used to give further protection. Some of the covers designed specifically for incontinence have antifungal and antibacterial layers. Waterproof covers for duvets and pillows are also available.

To protect chairs, absorbent waterproof chair pads and cushion covers are available. Like bed pads, they may be washable or disposable.

Faecal incontinence

Many people have an occasional temporary loss of faecal continence when they suffer from a bout of severe diarrhoea (p.171). Severe, long-term constipation can also cause faecal incontinence if the rectum becomes overfull with a solid faecal mass and fluid and small pieces of faeces leak out around the mass. However, there are many other possible causes of faecal incontinence, and therefore it is important to consult a doctor if the person you are caring for experiences it persistently or repeatedly.

Dealing with faecal incontinence

If the person's incontinence is associated with constipation or diarrhoea, it may be possible to control it by adjusting the person's diet. In general, a high-fibre diet is better for constipation-associated incontinence and a low-fibre diet for diarrhoea-associated incontinence. However, you should consult a doctor about specific recommendations for the person in your care. The doctor will also be able

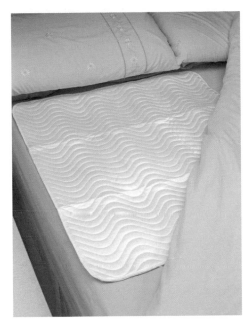

Bed protector
Pads to protect the bed have an absorbent top layer with a waterproof backing. Disposable and reusable, washable versions are available.

to advise about any medications or other treatments that may be appropriate.

In some cases, it may be possible to improve continence with pelvic floor exercises (p.137) or with bowel retraining, which involves establishing a regular time for the person to open her bowels and also finding specific ways to stimulate bowel movements.

Many of the aids for urinary incontinence are also suitable for faecal incontinence, such as pads, pants, and bed and chair protectors, although it is usually better to choose disposable versions for faecal incontinence. The person may also find it helpful to use an anal plug. This is a piece of foam that is inserted into the anus and expands on contact with moisture, thereby preventing soiling. If in any doubt about the suitability of such aids, you should consult a doctor or continence advisor.

URINARY CATHETER CARE

A **urinary catheter** is a flexible sterile tube inserted into the bladder to drain urine into a collecting bag. The person may have two types of bag: a leg bag for daytime use and a larger night bag. Guidelines for catheter and bag care are outlined here. A health professional will provide more detailed information, and you should follow that if it differs from the advice given here.

Routine care

A crucial aspect of caring for a person who has a urinary catheter is maintaining good hygiene to pevent infection (see panel, right). You should also encourage the person to have a bath or shower every day, and to drink at least 1.5–2l (2.5–3.5 pints) of fluid a day.

The catheter and leg bag should be secured firmly to the person's body, and the leg bag should be emptied before it gets too full in order to prevent pulling. The leg bag should be changed only every week, or if it gets damaged or dirty.

The night bag should be supported by the side of the person's bed, off the floor and below the level of the bladder. The

night bag should be changed every week, or if it gets damaged or dirty.

When emptying a leg bag or night bag, do not let the outlet spout touch the floor or the rim of the toilet or container. After the bag has been emptied, clean the outlet spout with an alcohol wipe and close the end of the spout securely.

When to seek medical help

Seek immediate medical help if the person has any of the following: fever, vomiting, unusual confusion or tiredness, pain in the lower back or near the bladder, blood in the urine, or offensive-smelling urine. If the catheter comes out or if there are any problems you don't know how to deal with, contact a doctor or health professional.

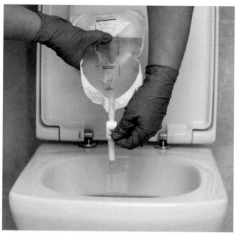

Emptying a drainage bag

Drainage bags should be emptied into a clean toilet or container. Every time you empty the person's bag, wear a new pair of sterile gloves.

STOMA CARE

A stoma is an opening made in the wall of the abdomen to allow wastes to empty into a bag on the surface of the skin. A stoma may be temporary or permanent and is created surgically after an operation such as a colostomy or ileostomy. A colostomy creates a stoma from the large intestine, enabling wastes to pass out without going through the anus. An ileotomy creates a stoma from the small intestine, allowing wastes to pass out without going through the large intestine. A stoma may also be created after a urostomy, allowing urine to pass out without going through the bladder, but this procedure is relatively uncommon and is not covered here.

After the operation, a specialist stoma nurse will teach you how to care for the stoma, how to obtain new bags and other supplies, and will advise about aspects of daily living such as diet. The information given here is primarily a reminder of the key points of stoma care after a colostomy or ileostomy.

Routine care

Because waste passes out through the stoma, it is important to keep the skin around it clean. The area should be washed every time the bag is changed. It should be cleaned gently with water and dry wipes or clean, soft paper towel. Do not use harsh soaps or disinfectants as these may irritate the skin. Do not rub the stoma too hard as stomas tend to bleed easily, but don't worry if there is a small amount of bleeding from the outside surface of the stoma as this should stop quite quickly.

■ **Changing a stoma bag** There are different types of stoma bag and the details of how and when to change them vary. The guidelines below apply to most types of bag, but the stoma nurse will give you specific instructions on how and when to change the bag for the person in your care.

Before changing the bag, assemble all the items you will need and ensure there is sufficient privacy. Remove the bag, working gently from the top to the bottom of the flange (the part that sticks to the skin). When removing the bag, you may need to use medical adhesive remover to avoid damaging the skin. Wash the area around the stoma and dry it thoroughly with dry wipes or clean, soft paper towel. If the person is susceptible to sore skin, use barrier wipes, spray, or lotion around the stoma. When the skin is dry, fit the new bag, making sure it is secure all the way round.

When to seek medical help

Usually, a stoma causes few problems once the person and you as the carer become used to managing it. However, you should contact the stoma nurse if the skin around the stoma becomes inflamed or bleeds persistently, if blood is coming out from inside the stoma, or if part of the intestine protrudes through the stoma. You can also contact the nurse even if all you need is advice about some aspect of stoma care.

EQUIPMENT FOR CHANGING A BAG

When changing a stoma bag, gather the necessary items beforehand. The items you may need are:

■ A new bag.

■ A plastic bag for the used stoma bag.

■ Medical adhesive remover.

■ Warm water.

■ Dry wipes or clean, soft paper towel.

■ Barrier wipes, spray, or lotion if the person is prone to soreness around the stoma.

8

DAY-TO-DAY
NURSING

■ BASIC SKILLS AND PRINCIPLES ■ USEFUL EQUIPMENT
■ MONITORING A PERSON'S CONDITION ■ KEY DANGER SIGNS
■ GIVING MEDICATION ■ WOUND CARE ■ PAIN MANAGEMENT
■ DEALING WITH TEMPERATURE PROBLEMS
■ DEALING WITH BREATHING PROBLEMS
■ DEALING WITH VOMITING AND DIARRHOEA

BASIC SKILLS AND PRINCIPLES

Whether you are new to caring for somebody at home or already have experience as a carer, this section will provide you with advice and guidance about practical nursing skills you may need. You will also be able to get assistance from your local community or district nursing services; your GP will be able to tell you how to access such help.

Good nursing practice

At the heart of good nursing practice is communication, both with the person you are caring for and with any health professionals. Any carer must treat somebody in their care with dignity and understanding, show compassion and sensitivity to their needs and wishes, and provide care in a respectful way. As the carer, it is important that you take advice from health professionals and, if possible, involve the person you are caring for in any decisions so that, together, you make agreed, informed choices. It is also important to work closely with health professionals to make sure you are using the best and most appropriate techniques and to ensure that any health risks are identified and managed properly. Two of the other cornerstones of good nursing practice are hygiene and organization, which are discussed below

Hygiene

Good hygiene is essential to prevent germs, such as bacteria, viruses, and fungi, from spreading, either directly from person to person or indirectly from touching contaminated surfaces or equipment. Ways to prevent such cross-infection include effective handwashing, using gloves and aprons, using and disposing of needles and other sharp implements (known as "sharps") safely, and cleaning and disinfecting equipment correctly.

Regular, careful handwashing is one of the most important ways of reducing the spread of infection. If the correct technique is used, washing your hands with soap and running water is usually sufficient (although antibacterial hand gel can be used in addition). However, germs are transferred more easily from wet hands, so it is also essential to dry your hands thoroughly afterwards. You should wash your hands before and after carrying out any nursing procedure, as well as before and after other activities, such as preparing or serving food.

A health professional may provide you with special gloves to be used as a

---

PROTECTING YOURSELF FROM INFECTION

It is important to protect yourself from infection, otherwise you may become ill yourself and be unable to continue to provide care. The measures described below can help to prevent you from getting an infection.

- Wash and dry your hands thoroughly before and after carrying out any nursing task.
- Cover any cuts or open skin you may have with a waterproof dressing.
- Avoid needlestick injury by taking care when using sharps and by putting them in a special sharps' container after use.
- Wear protective, disposable gloves and aprons when dealing with body fluids. Use disposable cloths and cleaning equipment if possible.
- Wash soiled linen or clothes at a temperature of 60°C (150°F) or above.
- Dispose of soiled dressings or pads by double-bagging them in plastic bags.
- If any body fluids get in your eyes or mouth, immediately flush them with copious amounts of clean water.

CORRECT HANDWASHING TECHNIQUE

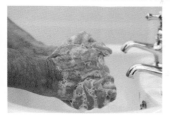

1 Wet your hands with water, making sure soap covers all your hand surfaces, and rub your palms together.

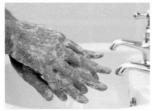

2 Rub the back of each hand with the palm of the other hand, with your fingers interlaced.

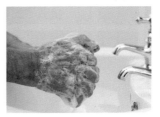

3 Put the palms of your hands together, interlace your fingers, and rub your palms together.

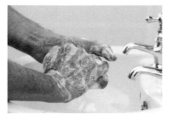

4 Interlock your fingers and rub the backs of your fingers with the palms of the opposite hand.

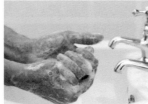

5 Clasp your thumb and rub it against your palm with a rotational movement. Clean each thumb in turn.

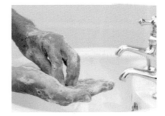

6 Rub your fingertips against your palm in a circular motion. Clean each hand in turn, rinse, and dry.

protective barrier. The gloves are usually made of latex, but if you or the person you're caring for is sensitive to latex, the health professional will be able to provide an alternative. You should also wear a disposable apron if there is a risk of contact with body fluids. Gloves and aprons should be disposed of properly, as advised by the health professional.

Sharps should be discarded immediately after use in an appropriate sharps container. Do not put this container in with the normal domestic waste but dispose of it as recommended by the health professional.

Clean surfaces and equipment regularly and thoroughly, using disposable cloths if possible. If reusable cloths are used, wash these after each use at a temperature of at least 60°C (150°F). Soiled clothing or bed linen should also be washed immediately at 60°C (150°F) or above. Wash mops and floor cloths in warm, soapy water, and disinfect and dry them after each use.

Organization

Good organization helps you to carry out tasks more efficiently and minimizes stress for you and the person you are caring for. To minimize disruption, coordinate nursing procedures with other tasks, such as changing bed linen, and set aside a specific time for such tasks, making sure they don't coincide with any prearranged visits.

Before carrying out any nursing task, ensure the environment is suitable and at the correct temperature, that there is sufficient privacy, and that the person will be comfortable. Make sure that all necessary equipment and medications are to hand, and check that the equipment is working properly.

USEFUL EQUIPMENT

As a home carer, you will find a general medical kit useful in helping you to carry out nursing tasks effectively, and it will also help you to deal with any medical problems that require first aid. You may need additional, more specialized pieces of equipment specifically for the person in your care. If so, contact your GP or ask a health professional for advice.

Home medical kit

A home medical kit is essentially the same as a first aid kit. You can make up your own or buy a ready-made kit and, if necessary, add to it so that it meets the needs of the person you are caring for as well as everybody living in your home. Your home medical kit should include:

- A first aid guide (see also the first aid section on pp.172–189 for help in dealing with medical emergencies).
- Washproof, hypoallergenic adhesive dressings in assorted sizes.

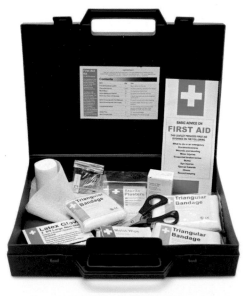

PORTABLE FIRST AID KIT

A portable first aid kit is useful for when you are out. Items to include in it are:

- Washproof, hypoallergenic adhesive dressings.
- Non-adhesive wound dressings.
- A crepe bandage and safety pins.
- A triangular bandage.
- A resuscitation mask.
- Sterile gauze swabs.
- Eye wash and a sterile eye pad.
- Disposable gloves and apron.
- Any prescribed medications, including emergency medications such as an EpiPen.
- Specialized items such as colostomy bags.
- A heat-retaining blanket.

- Thick, absorbent, non-adhesive surgical pads in sizes small, medium, and large; two of each size.
- Non-adhesive, dry-wound dressings in sizes small, medium, and large; two of each size.
- Adhesive transparent dressings; five medium size.
- Tubular bandages with applicators in assorted sizes.
- Three triangular bandages for slings.
- Crepe or other bandages to secure dressings.
- Five sterile gauze swabs for cleaning wounds.
- Five sterile cleansing wipes.
- Eye wash and two sterile eye pads.
- Microporous tape for securing dressings.
- Six safety pins for securing bandages.

First aid kit

A ready-made first aid kit will provide most of the items you need and can be supplemented with any extra items you require.

Two cool packs for sprains and bruises; keep the packs refrigerated.
- Blunt scissors.
- Tweezers.
- Disposable gloves.
- A thermometer (see p.148 for more information about thermometers).
- A resuscitation mask.

Medications to keep at home include:
- Painkillers (paracetamol and ibuprofen).
- Antiseptic cream or gel.
- Antihistamine tablets.

Make sure that all medications are within their use-by dates, and do not give more than the recommended dose. Check with the doctor of the person you are caring for whether the person should avoid any non-prescribed medications, including any complementary remedies.

Other equipment

Other items you may find useful include disposable aprons; clinical waste bags; incontinence pads; sheet protectors; a sharps' container; antiseptic liquid; general cleaning wipes; antibacterial hand gel; mouth swabs; bowls for vomit and for personal hygiene; and extra towels. You may also need items for giving oral medications, such as measuring spoons, cups, and oral syringes. A pill organizer, or dosette, box (p.159), can be useful if the person you are caring for needs to take several medications.

More specialized items that may be useful or necessary include syringe driver bags, which allow a person to walk around while medication is being administered via a syringe driver; a blood pressure monitor (p.149); and, if the person has diabetes, a blood glucose monitor (p.151). A health professional will be able to advise about the types and use of such items.

Safe storage

Your home medical kit should be kept in a cool, dry place, out of the reach of children but still easily accessible. All medicines should be kept in a separate, locked medicine cabinet.

SPECIAL DRESSINGS

There are many different types of special dressings. The types shown below are those you are likely to find most useful when caring for somebody at home.

- Thick, absorbent surgical pads are used to place over existing dressings when fluid is leaking through. They are non-adhesive and should be secured with microporous tape.

- Non-adhesive dry dressings are used to cover dry wounds or other specialist dressings.

- Adhesive transparent dressings are used to cover and protect wounds and blood-vessel catheter sites.

- Tubular bandages are placed over existing dressings to keep them in place.

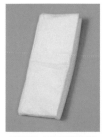

THICK, ABSORBENT SURGICAL PAD

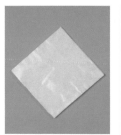

NON-ADHESIVE DRY DRESSING

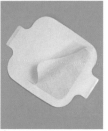

ADHESIVE TRANSPARENT DRESSING

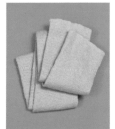

TUBULAR BANDAGE

MONITORING A PERSON'S CONDITION

An important aspect of home care is being aware of the person's health so that you notice any change and can, if necessary, take appropriate action. You may also have been asked by the person's doctor or other health professional to record the person's vital signs. These include breathing, body temperature, blood pressure, pulse, and, if the person has diabetes, blood sugar levels. Before taking any of these measurements, it is important that the person is calm, rested, and has not recently exerted himself.

Checking breathing

Most people change their breathing rate when they know that it is being measured. To get an accurate measurement, the person should therefore be unaware that his breathing rate is being counted. One way of doing this is to measure the breathing rate immediately after you have taken the person's pulse (pp.150–151). Keep your fingers on the person's wrist but, instead of counting the pulse, count the number of breaths you see as his chest rises and falls. If it is difficult to see the chest movements, place your hand lightly on the person's stomach to feel it rise and fall. The breathing rate is the number of breaths per minute, so you need to count them for a full 60 seconds to get an accurate measurement.

As well as checking the breathing rate, you should also look out for changes in the quality of the person's breathing – whether he has started wheezing, for instance. Because everybody is different, discuss with the person's doctor or other health professional what is normal for the person and what to look out for. If the

quality of breathing changes, note the changes and and inform the doctor or health professional, because they may indicate a respiratory problem.

Taking body temperature

There are several ways of measuring temperature. The most familiar is the oral (mouth) method, but it can also be measured aurally (in the ear), in the armpit, or on the forehead. It may be useful to discuss the most suitable method for your specific needs with the person's doctor or health professional, who will also be able to advise about which type of thermometer to use. Mercury thermometers are no longer available and should not be used; if you have one, you should dispose of it safely. Unless you are using a disposable, single-use thermometer, you should make sure the thermometer has been cleaned before every use (see panel, opposite).

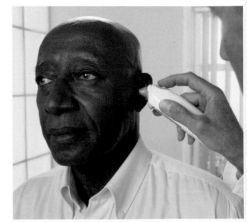

Using an aural thermometer
An aural thermometer should be placed gently in the outer ear canal and left in place until it beeps, after which the reading can be taken.

■ **Oral method** Place the thermometer under the person's tongue for about 2–3 minutes (the exact time may vary, depending on the specific model), making sure that the person keeps his mouth closed. Then remove the thermometer and note the reading. If the person has just eaten or drunk something hot or cold, wait for 10 minutes before taking his temperature.

■ **Aural method** Place the thermometer in the person's ear by using a gentle rocking motion until it sits comfortably in the ear canal. Wait until the thermometer beeps – which typically takes a few seconds – then remove it and note the reading. Body temperature measured in the ear gives the same reading as when it is measured in the mouth.

■ **Armpit method** Put the thermometer high up in the person's armpit and gently hold his arm against his body to ensure the skin is in direct contact with the thermometer. Leave the thermometer in place for as long as recommended in the instructions, then remove it and note the

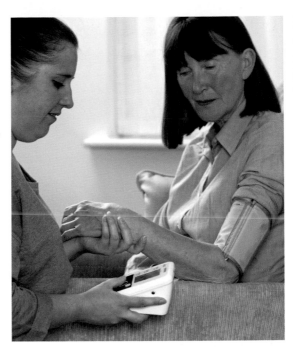

Using a blood pressure monitor
Place the cuff snugly around the upper arm and press the start button. The cuff will inflate, then deflate, and the monitor will display the readings.

reading from the digital display. Be aware that body temperature measured under the armpit is about 0.5°C (1°F) lower than body temperature measured orally.

■ **Forehead method** Place a thermometer strip on the person's forehead and leave it for as long as recommended in the instructions before reading off the temperature. Thermometer strips are not accurate, because they measure skin temperature rather than body temperature, but they can give an indication of whether a person is too hot or too cold.

Checking blood pressure

A person's blood pressure can be easily affected by a wide variety of factors, such as nervousness and activity level, so when you are checking blood pressure, it is important to make sure the person

---

CLEANING A THERMOMETER

Apart from single-use thermometers, all thermometers should be cleaned before and after every use.

■ Wash the thermometer in lukewarm, soapy water, rinse in cool, clean water, then dry thoroughly with a clean cloth or paper towel.

■ Alternatively, clean the thermometer with an alcohol wipe, rinse in cool, clean water, then dry thoroughly with a clean cloth or paper towel.

■ If the thermometer is not going to be used immediately, store it in a cool, dry place, out of the reach of children.

» MONITORING A PERSON'S CONDITION

remains rested and calm during the entire procedure. Also, to get an accurate reading, you should take the measurement from the same arm and at roughly the same time of day.

Blood pressure is usually measured with a digital blood pressure monitor. There are two main types: one with a cuff that fits around the wrist, the other with a cuff that fits around the upper arm. The latter is usually recommended, because it is generally more accurate than the wrist-cuff type. The instructions given below are for the type with an upper-arm cuff.

■ **Taking a measurement** Once you have made sure the person is relaxed and rested, roll up or remove his sleeve. Make sure the person's arm is supported so that the blood pressure cuff is level with his heart; you may need to use pillows to support the arm in the correct position. Slide the cuff on to the arm, making sure it sits about 2–3cm (1 inch) above the bend of the elbow. Fasten the cuff snugly and press the start button on the monitor. The cuff will first inflate then deflate, and the blood pressure measurements will appear on the monitor's screen. Two figures are shown: the higher figure is called the systolic pressure and is the blood pressure when the heart contracts to pump blood; the lower figure is called the diastolic pressure and is the blood pressure when the heart relaxes between contractions. Many blood pressure

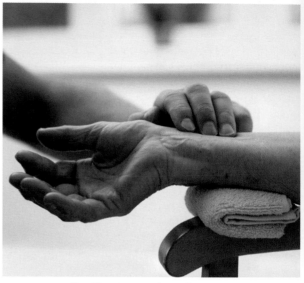

Checking the wrist (radial) pulse
With the person's arm supported in a relaxed position, place three fingers below the thumb and count the pulses in one minute.

monitors also show the pulse rate, which is the same as the number of heartbeats per minute.

You should measure the person's blood pressure as often as the health professional recommends, and keep a record of the readings.

Checking the pulse

The pulse is the rhythmic expansion and contraction of an artery as blood is pumped through it by the heart. It can be felt at many places on the body, where an artery crosses over a bone and is close to the skin's surface, such as the wrist or neck.

■ **Taking the pulse**. When you are checking a person's pulse, he should be relaxed and rested. Do not use your thumb, because it has a noticeable pulse of its own and it can be difficult to tell the difference between the person's pulse and your own. Instead, use your first three fingers.

The radial pulse in the wrist is probably the easiest to take. Place your first three fingers on the inside of the person's wrist just below the thumb. Press lightly until you can feel the rhythmic beats of the pulse under the skin. If you can't feel anything at first, apply a little pressure or slightly reposition your fingers.

If you can't find a pulse at the wrist, you can try the carotid pulse in the neck instead. Press lightly with your first and middle fingers on the side of the person's neck in the soft hollow area on the outside of his windpipe. Make sure you do not press too hard as this may make the person feel dizzy or light-headed.

When you have found a pulse, use a clock or watch with a second hand to count how many pulses there are in 60 seconds to give the pulse rate. You can also check if the pulse is regular or not. As with other measurements, record your findings.

Checking blood sugar

If the person you are caring for has diabetes, you may be asked by a health professional to monitor his blood sugar

(also known as blood glucose) levels on a regular basis. The health professional will tell you how frequently such monitoring needs to be done. However, you should check the blood sugar level more often if the person is unwell, and you should

USING A BLOOD SUGAR METER

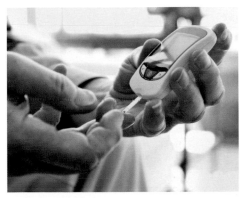

1 Before obtaining a blood sample from the person, his hands should be washed in warm water and dried. Gently squeeze the tip of one of the person's fingers, and use a sterile lancet to prick the fingertip and obtain a small drop of blood. It is less painful to prick the side, rather than the middle, of the fingertip and to use a different finger each time.

2 Place the drop of blood on the test strip and insert the strip into the monitor. The monitor will automatically measure the blood sugar level and display the reading. Record the result and clean off any excess blood from the person's finger using a sterile wipe.

» MONITORING A PERSON'S CONDITION

also make additional checks if you think he has any symptoms of low blood sugar (hypoglycaemia) or high blood sugar (hyperglycaemia).

Symptoms of hypoglycaemia (a "hypo") include dizziness, confusion, sweating, and shaking. It is potentially life-threatening and requires immediate action (see Dealing with hypoglycaemia, previous page). If you are unsure whether the person you are caring for is having a hypo, do not hesitate to get urgent medical help.

Symptoms of hyperglycaemia include an altered level of consciouness such as confusion or sleepiness, blurred vision, frequent urination, and excessive thirst. If the person you are caring for has any of these symptoms and his blood sugar level is higher than advised by his doctor or other health professional, get prompt medical advice.

■ **Measuring blood sugar** The most common method of measuring blood sugar is to use a special blood sugar meter. There are various types available, but they all work by analysing the amount of sugar in a

blood sample placed on a test strip inserted in the meter. The blood sample is obtained by using a lancet, a cutting device with a double blade. The illustrations on the previous page explain how to use one of the common types of blood glucose meter, but you should follow the manufacturer's instructions for your specific model. Before getting a blood glucose meter, ask a health professional for advice about the type most suitable for the person in your care.

Checking the skin
An essential part of looking after somebody at home is checking the skin. You should check for any rashes, and also for sore areas (such as pressure, or bed, sores) and broken skin.

Simply asking the person if he has noticed any skin problems is a good first step. However, this may not always be feasible – for example, if he has dementia – or he may not be aware of any problems on areas that are difficult to see, such as the back. Therefore make sure you also regularly check the person's skin yourself. This can often be done during routine tasks, such as personal hygiene or changing the bed linen. Before carrying out a skin check, make sure the environment is comfortable and has sufficient privacy.

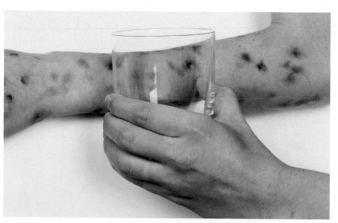

Glass test for meningitis rash
Press a glass tumbler against the rash. If the rash does not fade under pressure, this could be an indication of meningitis.

Because of the intimate nature of such a check, it is essential that it is done in such a way as to preserve the person's dignity.

If the person has a rash together with shortness of breath, swelling of the face, and tightness in the throat, he may be suffering from a severe allergic reaction called anaphylactic shock. This is a potentially life-threatening condition and requires immediate action: call an ambulance and see p.187.

Another type of rash to look out for specifically is the meningitis rash. Tiny pink spots appear and develop rapidly into dark red or purple blotches that resemble small bruises. They can appear anywhere on the body and do not fade when pressed; you can check this by using the glass text (see opposite). If the person develops such a rash, call an ambulance. If you find any other type of rash and there is no obvious cause for it (such as heat), seek medical advice.

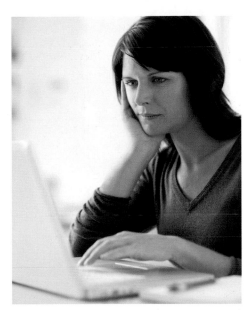

Recording health information
When recording information, make sure it is well organized and intelligible so that it can be readily understood when referred to later.

Checking mental status

It is just as important to be aware of the mental state of the person you are caring for as it is to monitor his physical wellbeing. Keeping such a check on the person's mental condition can be done informally, as part of your normal daily interactions. You may notice that the person is unhappy, withdrawn, or has lost interest in things he previously enjoyed. Or there may be changes such as memory loss, problems thinking, or finding it hard to follow conversations. There are many possible causes for such changes, so if you notice that the person's mental wellbeing has deteriorated, you should contact the person's doctor. In more extreme cases, the person may become extremely confused and/or agitated or may even become less than fully conscious of his surroundings. If any of these signs develop, get urgent medical help.

Record-keeping

With a busy life as a carer, record-keeping can be seen as a last priority. However, accurate health records of the person you are caring for will give health professionals valuable data that will enable them to monitor the person's condition and, if necessary, adjust treatment.

As well as recording health data, it is important to record details of the person's medication and any allergies he may have. It is also useful to keep notes concerning his preferences about such things as food, bathing times, favourite television programmes, and so on. These will be useful in helping to maintain the established routine if somebody else takes over caring from you while you have a break.

KEY DANGER SIGNS

Any person's health can deteriorate at any time. It is therefore important that you are able to recognize health problems in the person you are caring for promptly so that you can take the appropriate action. The chart below lists some of the key danger signs and the action required. However, if the person shows any other signs of illness or deterioration in his condition and you are uncertain about what to do, do not hesitate to seek medical advice.

SIGNS AND ACTION

SIGNS	ACTION
Difficulty breathing or breathlessness	■ If the person is choking, see p.178. ■ Admininster any medication prescribed for a breathing problem and seek medical advice. If medication is ineffective, call an ambulance. ■ In all other cases, call an ambulance.
Unexplained chest pain	■ Reassure the person and help him into a position that is comfortable. ■ Administer any medication prescribed for chest pain and seek medical advice. If medication is ineffective, call an ambulance. ■ If the person stops breathing, see p.176.
Facial drooping, limb weakness, difficulty speaking	■ Call an ambulance. ■ Put the person in the recovery position (see First aid, p.175) and give constant reassurance until medical help arrives.
Impaired consciousness	■ If the person is totally unconscious, see p.175. ■ If the person is partly conscious and has diabetes, see panel on p.151. ■ If the person is partly conscious and has been prescribed oxygen, administer the oxygen and call an ambulance. ■ In all other cases, call an ambulance.
Sudden facial swelling associated with breathing difficulty and itchy rash	■ If you suspect the person is having a severe allergic reaction (anaphylaxis), see p.187. ■ In all other cases, call an ambulance. Give constant reassurance until medical help arrives.
Vomiting blood	■ Call an ambulance. ■ Give the person a bowl for the vomit. Keep a sample of vomit for medical personnel. ■ Give the person a damp cloth to wipe his face. Do not give him fluids to drink. Instead, offer ice cubes to remove any unpleasant taste in his mouth.

GIVING MEDICATION

Giving medication safely is an important part of your role as a carer. It will help if you understand why you are giving a particular medication and how and when to give it, as well as any possible side effects or interactions with other medications and any special dietary advice. Because of the possibility of interactions or side effects, it is essential that you give only medications (including non-prescription drugs and complementary remedies) that have been prescribed or approved by the person's doctor.

Forms of medication

Medication can come in a wide variety of different forms. The more common ones include tablets, capsules, oral liquids, lozenges, powders, sprays, eye- and eardrops, lotions and other topical liquids, creams, gels, ointments, patches, pessaries, suppositories, and liquids for injection or catheter administration. Medication can also be administered by different methods and routes, such as orally (by mouth), by inhalation, topically to the skin, eyes, ears, or nose, via the rectum or vagina, by injection, and through a catheter inserted through the skin. The forms of medication and methods of administration covered below are those you are most likely to encounter when caring for somebody at home.

Administering medication

A few "golden rules" apply when giving any medication: make sure you are giving the right medication, to the right person, at the right dose, by the right route, and at the right time. You should also read the information leaflet. Before administering any medication, always explain to the person what you are going to give him.

HANDLING DRUGS SAFELY

When giving drugs to the person you are caring for, you should avoid direct skin contact with the drugs. If you spill a liquid on yourself, wash it off at once with plenty of water. In the unlikely event that you develop any unusual symptoms, seek medical advice.

Handling drugs
Some drugs can be absorbed through the skin. To avoid getting a dose yourself, use disposable gloves when handling them.

Administering oral medication

Giving drugs by mouth is the most common method of administration. If the medication is a pill to be swallowed, you should offer water with the pill. If swallowing pills is a problem, your doctor may be able to prescribe the drug in a different form. Do not crush pills to make them easier to swallow without first consulting a doctor, because some pills must be swallowed whole. Some oral medication is designed to be placed in the mouth but not swallowed. If the person has been prescribed this type, make sure he is aware that it must not be swallowed.

If the medication is in liquid form, shake the bottle well and pour the required dose into a measuring cup on a flat, level surface. The person may find it easier

›› GIVING MEDICATION

to take the medication from a syringe. If so, direct the syringe towards the inside of the person's cheek near the back of his mouth and administer the medication in small squirts.

Administering inhaled medication

Inhaled medications are used primarily for respiratory conditions, such as asthma, and are most commonly administered via an inhaler or nebulizer.

There are many different types of inhaler, and it is important that you know the correct way of using the type prescribed for the person in your care. A nebulizer is a machine that turns liquid medication into a fine mist that can be inhaled easily through a facemask or mouthpiece. Whether the person you are caring for uses an inhaler or nebulizer, a health professional will give you the necessary instructions about how to use the equipment properly. There is also more information in Dealing with breathing problems (pp.166–167).

Administering topical skin medication

Topical skin medications come in a variety of forms – creams, ointments, gels, lotions, and sprays, for example. Applied directly to

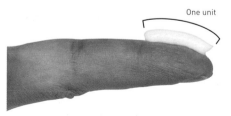

One unit

A fingertip unit
The fingertip unit can help you work out how much medication is needed to cover an area of skin. One unit is the amount that can be squeezed in a line to the first joint of the index finger; it will cover an area the size of both sides of one hand.

the skin's surface, they are used mainly to treat conditions such as dry skin, skin infections, and inflammatory conditions such as dermatitis. Some painkillers are also available as topical preparations.

Before you apply any topical medication, make sure there is sufficient privacy and that the person is comfortable. Wash and dry your hands, then put on a pair of disposable gloves, and clean and dry the affected area of the person's skin. Shake the container if the medication is a spray or lotion, then apply the medication as instructed by the person's doctor or other health professional or according to the instructions on the information sheet. Do not cover the area with a dressing unless instructed otherwise by the doctor or health professional. Finally, remove the disposable gloves, and wash and dry your hands.

Administering topical eye, ear, and nose medication

Medications applied directly to the eye, ear, or nose are used to treat conditions such as eye infections (for example, bacterial conjunctivitis) and itchy eyes; infections of the outer ear canal and excess earwax; and nasal congestion and hayfever.

■ **Eye medications** Before you administer any eye medication, wash and dry your hands. Make sure the person is sitting or reclining, then tilt his head back and gently pull down his eyelid. Tell the person to look upwards and then administer the prescribed number of drops or apply a thin line of ointment on the inside of his lower eyelid, making sure the nozzle of the medication bottle does not touch the eye. Gently release the lower eyelid and encourage the person to close his eye for a few seconds. Some eye medications

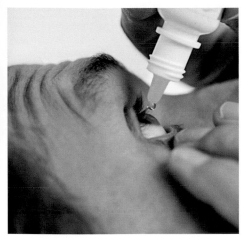

Administering eyedrops
Tilt the person's head back and draw his lower eyelid away from his eye. Drop the eyedrops on the inside of his lower eyelid.

can cause blurry vision, so make sure the person does not get up until his vision has cleared.

■ **Ear medications** Eardrops are best administered with the person lying down on his side. Before administering the drops, warm the dropper bottle in your hand for a few minutes, then gently squeeze the prescribed number of drops into the person's ear canal, ensuring that the dropper nozzle does not touch his ear. The person should remain lying down for a few minutes afterwards to ensure the medication does not run out of his ear.

■ **Nasal medications** These medications come in two main forms – drops and sprays – which are administered in different ways.

To administer drops, gently tilt the person's head back, drop the prescribed number of drops into each nostril in turn, then bend the person's head forwards and gently move it from side to side to distribute the medication evenly.
To administer spray, tilt the person's head forwards slightly and close one nostril by

gently pressing on the side of his nose. Insert the spray into the other nostril and tell the person to breathe in through his nose. While he is breathing in, squirt the spray into his nostril. Repeat for the other nostril, then tilt the person's head back so that the medication reaches the top of his nose.

Administering pessaries and suppositories

Pessaries and suppositories are plugs or capsules that are inserted into the vagina or rectum, respectively. They are designed to melt at body temperature, thereby releasing the medication they contain. Before administering a pessary or suppository, make sure that there is sufficient privacy and that the person knows exactly what you are going to do.

■ **Pessaries** Before administering a vaginal pessary, wash and dry your hands, put on disposable gloves, and unwrap the pessary. Ask the person to lie on her back with her legs open, or on her side with her top leg bent upwards towards her chest. Place lubricating gel on the pessary and then use your finger or an applicator to gently insert the pessary into the vagina as far as comfortably possible. Remove your finger or, if you are using an applicator, press the plunger to release the pessary into the vagina, then remove the applicator. Discard the gloves (and applicator, if you used one) and wash your hands.

■ **Suppositories** Before administering a rectal suppository, ask the person to empty his bowels and bladder. Then wash and dry your hands, put on disposable gloves, and unwrap the suppository. Ask the person to lie on his side, with both knees bent and drawn up towards his chest. Put a disposable incontinence sheet under the person's hips and buttocks in case the suppository is ejected prematurely or the person has an uncontrollable bowel movement immediately after the suppository has been inserted. It is also a wise precaution idea to have a bedpan or commode nearby. Place lubricating gel on the suppository and gently lift up the cheek of the top buttock so that you can see the rectum. Using one finger, carefully insert the suppository through the muscular sphincter of the rectum until it is about 2.5cm (1 inch) inside. After you have inserted the suppository, wipe away any excess lubricating gel. Encourage the person to remain lying on his side and to hold in the suppository for at least 15 minutes or until he is no longer able to do so, in order to give the medication time to be absorbed. Discard the disposable gloves and incontinence sheet, and wash your hands.

Administering injected medication

Injectable medications are made up in sterile solutions that come in vials, ampoules, bottles, cartridges, and preloaded injector pens. There are several different ways to inject medication, the most common being subcutaneously (under the skin) and intramuscularly (into

---

DEALING WITH NEEDLESTICK INJURY

You are unlikely to suffer a needlestick injury if you follow the correct procedure for giving injections (see main text, right). However, if you do accidentally stick yourself with a needle, follow the instructions below:

- Encourage the wound to bleed by holding it under warm, running water, then wash the area with soap and rinse under cool, running water.

- Dry the wound and cover it with a waterproof adhesive dressing.

- Seek urgent medical advice.

---

a muscle). Injectable medications can also be given intravenously (into a vein); this is usually done through a catheter or cannula (hollow tubes) inserted through the skin into a vein. Giving injected medication requires a certain amount of skill. If you need to administer injections, a health professional will ensure you receive proper instruction.

■ **Subcutaneous and intramuscular injections** A subcutaneous injection is given into the fatty tissue under the skin. Common injection sites include the back of the arms, the middle and outer areas of the thighs, the abdomen, and the buttocks. It is important to rotate the injection sites because repeated injections in the same place can cause tissue damage. An intramuscular injection is given into a muscle. Common injection sites include the upper arm, leg, and buttocks. Both of these types of injection are given using a needle and syringe, and the general technique is the same for both.

Before giving an injection, make sure the person is relaxed, explain what you are going to do, and make sure you have all the equipment you need. You will need the medication, a needle and syringe, alcohol swabs, a gauze swab, an adhesive dressing, disposable gloves, and a sharps' box. Wash and dry your hands and put on the disposable gloves. Wipe the person's skin with the alcohol swab, wait a few seconds for the alcohol to dry, then give the injection as you have been instructed. Wipe the area with the sterile gauze and apply a small adhesive dressing. Do not resheath the needle but dispose of it immediately in the sharps' box. Remove your gloves and wash and dry your hands.

■ **Intravenous injections and indwelling catheters** An intravenous injection is a

INDWELLING CATHETER MAINTENANCE

An indwelling catheter requires strict aseptic technique and careful maintenance.

- Wash and dry your hands and put on sterile gloves before handling the catheter.

- Use a sterile dressing to secure the catheter in place. Use a transparent dressing to enable you to check the insertion site for infection. Replace sterile dressings every seven days, or sooner if the dressing gets wet, is soiled, or is not securely in place.

- Check for signs of infection every day; such signs include swelling, redness, pain, or leakage of fluid from the insertion site.

- Clean the catheter as instructed and with the solution provided. The catheter should be flushed with normal saline before and after use to prevent any blockages.

- If you see signs of infection or if you suspect the catheter is blocked, contact a health professional immediately.

method of giving medication directly into a vein, usually through a catheter or cannula, which will be inserted by a health professional. If the person you are caring for requires long-term medication, an indwelling catheter may be inserted instead. This will be done in hospital, but after insertion the catheter can be used and cared for at home. An indwelling catheter requires careful maintenance and must be kept free of infection (see panel, left). When the person is taking a

shower or bathing, the catheter should be covered with a waterproof dressing. You should also make sure the catheter is protected from being accidentally pulled. Whether the person requires intravenous injections or has an indwelling catheter, a health professional will come to his home to administer the medication.

Organizing medication

If the person has to take many different medications, you need to ensure he takes the right medication at the right time. There are many different pill organizer systems to help with this, such as dosette boxes and bubble packs, and some of them even have built-in timers that beep as a reminder of when a medication is due to be taken. You may also find it useful to make your own medicine sheet listing the medications and their dosage, when they should be taken, and other information, such as whether a medication needs to be taken with food.

Disposing of medication

The best way to dispose of medicines is to return them to your pharmacy, preferably in their original packets. Do not dispose of them down the sink or toilet, because they could contaminate the water supply. Arrangements for disposing of a sharps' bin vary from area to area. A health professional will be able to advise about the arrangements in your specific area.

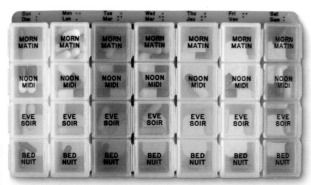

Pill organizer box
A pill, or dosette, box has sections for different days and different times of day, and is a handy way of making sure you administer the right medication at the right time.

159

WOUND CARE

If the person in your care has a wound, such as a skin ulcer or surgical incision, it is important to look after it properly to ensure that it does not become infected and that it heals well. The wound will need to be checked regularly. This is best done at the same time as changing the dressing, to make sure the wound is disturbed as little as possible. The information given here primarily concerns caring for wounds after they have been treated by a medical professional. First aid for wounds is given on p.180.

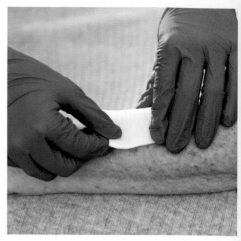

Applying a dressing to a small wound
After cleaning and drying a small wound, cover it with a non-adhesive dressing, then secure the dressing with a bandage or tape.

Changing a dressing

There are many different types of wound dressing, and a health professional will have chosen the appropriate one for the person's particular wound. If it is a specialized dressing, it will be changed by the health professional. If the person has an ordinary type of dressing, the health professional will teach you how to change it; he or she will also show you how to clean small wounds.

The techniques described here are suitable for most types of non-specialized dressings and small wounds, but you should follow the health professional's instructions if they differ from those given here. Before changing any dressing, you need to ensure that there is sufficient privacy and that the person is in a comfortable position.

■ **Removing the old dressing** Wash your hands thoroughly and put on a pair of sterile gloves. Open a sterile dressing pack as instructed by the health professional. Take off the existing dressing by gently removing any tape that is securing it to the person's skin – taking care not to pull the skin – and remove the dressing with sterile forceps. If the dressing is sticking

to the wound, wet the dressing with sterile water to loosen it.

■ **Checking the wound** Once you have removed the old dressing, check to see how well the wound is healing and for any signs of infection. It is normal for some wounds to weep a small amount of clear fluid for a short time, but if there is a large amount of fluid or if it is green or yellow in colour, the wound may be infected. Other signs of infection include redness, swelling, localized heat around the wound, and increasing pain in the wound; it may also have an offensive smell.

■ **Cleaning the wound** After checking the wound, it needs to be cleaned. Put on a new pair of sterile gloves and wipe the wound gently with sterile gauze and saline, or as instructed by the health professional. Clean the wound from the middle outwards, taking care not to disrupt healing tissue. Dry the surrounding skin with sterile gauze.

If the person has fragile skin, follow the guidelines below to help prevent skin tears:

- Use an emollient to keep the skin moist.
- Dry the skin by patting rather than rubbing.
- Encourage the person to wear clothing that covers as much skin as possible and is loose enough not to rub the skin.
- Protect fragile areas by covering them with loose tubular gauze.
- Handle the person gently, and take extra care when removing dressings that are secured with tape.

■ **Applying a new dressing** When the wound is clean and dry, cover it with a non-adhesive dressing and secure the dressing with a crepe bandage, a tubular bandage, or microporous tape.

Discard all used dressings and gloves in the clinical waste bag provided by the health professional, and thoroughly wash your hands. Make sure the person is comfortable, and note down any changes to the wound for reference.

■ **Specialized dressings** If the person has a specialized dressing, you should not change it and clean the wound yourself. The health professional will visit regularly to perform these tasks. However, you should check the dressing regularly to ensure that blood or other body fluids have not soaked through. If there has been leakage through the dressing, put a thick, absorbent, non-adhesive dressing on top and secure it with microporous tape. Then contact the health professional without delay.

Preventing infection

If a wound becomes infected, it may heal not heal properly, and there is also the possibility that the infection will spread and cause other health problems.

Making sure both you and the person you are caring for maintain high standards of personal hygiene is an essential basic step in preventing infection. Good wound-cleaning technique (see opposite) is also vital, as is keeping the dressing clean and dry. Make sure that the dressing is protected with a waterproof cover when the person bathes or showers. If the dressing becomes wet or soiled, change it immediately. You should also discourage the person from disturbing the dressing.

Other measures to help prevent infection include ensuring the person has a healthy diet, so that his immune system is strong, and keeping him as active as possible to encourage good blood flow to the wound. It is also important to ensure that any disorders that impair the immune system, such as diabetes, are well controlled.

When to get medical help

Contact the health professional immediately if the person's wound shows any signs of infection (see Checking the wound, opposite); if there are any problems with a specialized dressing; or if the person starts to feel generally unwell or develops symptoms such as a fever or swollen glands.

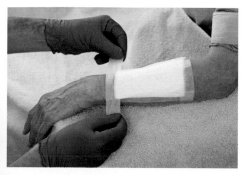

Applying a second dressing
If blood or other fluids have leaked through a specialized dressing, put a thick, absorbent dressing on top and secure it with tape.

PAIN MANAGEMENT

Pain is not only unpleasant itself but can also cause problems such as fatigue, emotional distress, and poor quality of life. There are two kinds of pain: acute pain, which comes on suddenly and lasts for a short time; and chronic pain, which is long-lasting. The information given here relates to chronic pain. If the person in your care is suffering from acute pain, you should contact the person's doctor. For chronic pain, make sure the person has a pain assessment by a pain specialist. Together, they will agree on a pain management plan for you to follow. This will often involve medication but may also include other methods, such as relaxation techniques, physiotherapy, or a TENS machine.

Pain medication

There are many drugs that can relieve pain (known as analgesics), and the most common are listed in the table below. Other drugs sometimes used to relieve pain include corticosteroids, used to treat inflammation, and certain antidepressants and anti-seizure medications, which can be effective for some cases of nerve pain.

Analgesics are most commonly given as pills, but they may also be administered by injection, by syringe driver (a pump that delivers medication continuously), by rectal suppository, or by skin patch. The pain specialist will advise on the most appropriate medication and method of administration for the person in your care. You should follow this advice carefully to ensure pain is controlled properly. Because the effects of analgesics gradually wear off, it is important to make sure they are given on time and at the correct dose.

Do not give the person any other, non-prescribed medications or complementary remedies without first consulting the person's doctor, because some may interact with other medications, some should not be used by people with certain conditions, and some contain analgesics, which may lead to an accidental overdose.

COMMON TYPES OF PAIN MEDICATION

TYPES	USES	COMMON SIDE EFFECTS
Opioids (e.g. codeine, fentanyl, morphine, tramadol)	Used to treat moderate to severe pain.	■ Drowsiness. ■ Constipation. ■ Nausea/vomiting. ■ Dizziness.
Nonsteroidal anti-inflammatory drugs (e.g. aspirin, diclofenac, ibuprofen)	Used to relieve mild to moderate pain and to reduce inflammation; asprin also reduces fever.	■ Heartburn/indigestion/ stomach irritation. ■ Nausea/vomiting.
Other painkillers (e.g. nefopam, paracetamol)	Used to relieve mild to moderate pain; paracetamol also reduces fever.	■ Nausea/vomiting. ■ Other side effects depend on the specific drug; see drug information leaflet.

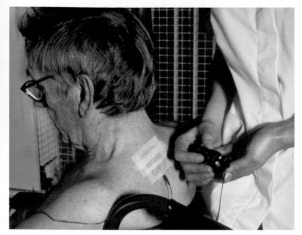

Using a TENS machine
Electrodes are attached to the skin in the area of pain, and the machine is turned on. Usually, the machine must be kept on for at least 45 minutes to produce any noticeable pain relief.

Other methods of pain relief

If medication by itself does not relieve pain, other methods can be tried in combination with medication or by themselves. Simple relaxation techniques are often helpful in managing pain. Physical exercises can

also be useful in some cases, particularly for muscle or joint pain. A physiotherapist will be able to advise you on the most suitable exercises for the person you are looking after.

The pain specialist may suggest using a TENS (transcutaneous electrical nerve stimulation) machine alongside pain medications. This device sends tiny electric currents through electrodes attached to the skin and is thought to work by blocking pain signals to the brain. It typically takes about 45–60 minutes for a TENS machine to produce pain relief, but it can usually be used for several hours at a time, several times a day. However, TENS machines cannot be used by everybody, so consult the pain specialist before buying one.

Other techniques that may be effective include acupuncture, meditation, and self-hypnosis. There is little proper medical evidence about the effectiveness of these techniques, but anecdotal reports suggest they may help in some cases.

In certain cases, more invasive treatment may be an option, such as an injection of anaesthetic (a nerve block), or even radiotherapy, chemotherapy, or surgery. The pain specialist or person's doctor will advise you if he or she thinks the person would benefit from any of these treatments.

When to get medical help

Consult the person's doctor or pain specialist if his pain gets worse and/or is no longer adequately controlled by medication or any other methods you have tried. You should also get prompt medical advice if the person experiences severe or unexpected side effects from any pain medication.

DEALING WITH BREAKTHROUGH PAIN

Breakthrough pain is a flare-up of pain between doses of medication or other forms of pain control. If the person experiences such pain, try the following:

- Administer any specific medication prescribed by the person's doctor for breakthrough pain.

- Try another form of pain control, such as relaxation exercises or a TENS machine.

- The person may find that simply changing position or resting alleviates the pain.

- If specific activities bring on breakthrough pain, administer any breakthrough medication beforehand.

- If breakthrough pain continues to be a problem, consult the pain specialist.

DEALING WITH TEMPERATURE PROBLEMS

The body can only function properly when its internal temperature is around 37ºC (98.6ºF). It is therefore important to monitor the temperature of the person you are caring for (pp.148–149). You also need to be aware of the signs of high and low temperature so you can recognize if the person's temperature is too high or low and can take the appropriate action.

Dealing with fever

A fever – generally defined as a body temperature above 38ºC (100.4ºF) – can cause a variety of different symptoms. These may include sweating, shivering, headache, muscle aches, general weakness, and loss of appetite. There is also a danger that the person may become dehydrated.

To lower the person's temperature and relieve symptoms, remove any excess

---

IMPORTANT!

Paracetamol and ibuprofen can help to reduce a fever but, before giving either of them to the person you are caring for, you must:

- Check with the person's doctor that they will not interact with any other medications the person is taking.

- Check that the person has not taken any other medications that contain paracetamol or ibuprofen (such as some over-the-counter painkillers, or cold and flu remedies) to ensure he does not accidentally take an overdose.

---

clothing he is wearing, making sure that there is sufficient privacy and the person's dignity is maintained. You should also encourage the person to rest and ensure that the room is well ventilated. Do not attempt to cool the person's skin directly – for example, by sponging with cool water – because this may cause him to shiver, which will increase his body temperature. To prevent the person from becoming dehydrated, encourage him to drink plenty of cool fluids. Paracetamol or ibuprofen can help to reduce fever, but see the panel (above) before giving either of these drugs to the person.

- **When to get medical help** A fever by itself may not be a cause for alarm or a reason to call a doctor. However, seek immediate medical

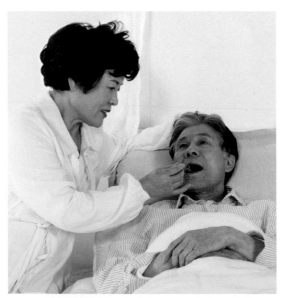

Checking body temperature
Body temperature can be checked easily with an oral thermometer (p.149). If it is too high or too low, you need to take corrective action immediately.

SIGNS OF HYPOTHERMIA

Hypothermia is a potentially fatal condition in which the body temperature falls below 35.5°C (96°F). The list below gives the signs that typically develop as hypothermia progresses. It is vital to treat hypothermia as early as possible (see p.188).

Early signs

- Feeling cold.
- Uncontrollable shivering.

Later signs

- Difficulty in concentrating and drowsiness.
- Dizziness and confusion.
- Slurred speech.
- Abnormally slow breathing or breathing difficulty.
- Finally, unconsciousness and death.

help if a fever worsens and/or lasts for more than 48 hours, or if the person's body temperature is 39.4°C (103°F) or higher. If the person has a fever and becomes confused, agitated, unresponsive, or has chest pain or difficulty breathing, call an ambulance. You should also call an ambulance if the person has a fever that is accompanied by a severe headache, a stiff neck, and/or a rash that does not fade when pressed (p.153) – these may be signs of meningitis, which is potentially life-threatening.

Dealing with low temperature

Low body temperature is a particular risk if the person's mobility is impaired, or if he is elderly or unwell. You should therefore take measures to prevent him from becoming cold and should also monitor his temperature so that you can take immediate action if it does fall too low.

■ **Preventing low body temperature** It is important to make sure the room the person is in is warm enough. You should ask the person about this, because the room temperature may seem warm enough to you but may not be for the person himself, especially if he is not moving around much. You should also check that he is not in a draught. Make sure that the person is dressed warmly enough or has sufficient bedding, and that extra clothing and/or bedding is within easy reach so that he can add more layers if he feels cold.

If you are going outside with the person, check the weather beforehand and ensure he is dressed appropriately. If the weather is cold, make sure he has a hot meal or drink before going out, and take extra clothing or blankets. You should also consider taking an insulated flask filled with a hot drink if you are intending to be out for a long time.

■ **Treating low body temperature** If, despite taking the preventive measures described above, the person complains of feeling cold or feels cold to the touch, you should take his temperature. If it is slightly below average for the person, you need to warm him up promptly. Warm up the room the person is in, or, if you are outside, move immediately to a warm environment. Help the person to put on more clothing and wrap him in blankets or a duvet, or add more bedding layers if he is in bed. If the person is fully conscious, give him a hot drink.

■ **When to get medical help** If the person's body temperature is slightly below average and the measures described above are unsuccessful, if symptoms progress (see panel, above), or if the person's body temperature falls below 35.5°C (96°F), call an ambulance and administer first aid for hypothermia (p.188).

DEALING WITH BREATHING PROBLEMS

There are many reasons why a person may have difficulty breathing or breathlessness. Some degree of breathlessness is normal after physical exercise, particularly in those who are unfit or overweight, and breathing difficulty due to nasal congestion is a common symptom of a common cold or flu. Emotional stress and anxiety can also sometimes cause breathlessness. The information given here provides practical advice for helping a person in your care who has breathing problems due to nasal congestion or who has previously been medically assessed and prescribed treatment for a breathing problem. In other cases, you should go straight to When to get medical help, p.169.

Relieving nasal congestion

Mild breathlessness due to nasal congestion can be treated easily with steam inhalation. When using this method, you should be careful to avoid scalding.

To prepare a steam inhalation, pour a few cups of boiling water into a large, shallow bowl, then let it cool for a minute or two. Place the bowl on a level, flat, non-slippery surface, or place a thin towel or rubber mat under the bowl to prevent it slipping. Place a towel over the person's head and help him to lean forwards over the bowl. Encourage him to breathe deeply for about 10 minutes. This should help loosen the mucus and make it easier for him to clear the nasal passages.

If this method is too difficult for the person, it is possible to buy a steamer with a mask that fits over the mouth and nose. Alternatively, you can sit with him in a hot, steamy bathroom.

Steam inhalation can only help relieve the nasal congestion itself, rather than the underlying cause. If congestion is due to a respiratory infection or disorder, the person may also require treatment of the underlying condition, so you should consult the person's doctor if congestion does not clear up within a few days, gets worse, or is accompanied by other symptoms.

Medication

If the person has a respiratory disorder, he may require treatment with medication. Respiratory infections are usually treated with antibiotics. If the person has been prescribed antibiotics, it is important that he finishes the full course, even if the symptoms have cleared up, to ensure the infection has been eradicated. You should also make sure the antibiotics are administered correctly; for example, some should be taken with food, whereas others should be taken on an empty stomach. Although

Using a nebulizer
A nebulizer converts liquid medication into a mist that is inhaled through a facemask placed over the mouth and nose.

antibiotics do not usually cause side effects, they may cause diarrhoea and nausea in some people. If severe diarrhoea and/or nausea do develop, see pp.170–171 and consult the person's doctor.

If the person has a respiratory condition such as asthma, chronic obstructive pulmonary disease (COPD), emphysema, or lung cancer, he may have been prescribed medication that is inhaled, either from an inhaler or via a nebulizer.

■ **Using an inhaler** There are many types of inhaler, and it is important that the correct technique is used to ensure the person receives the full benefit of the

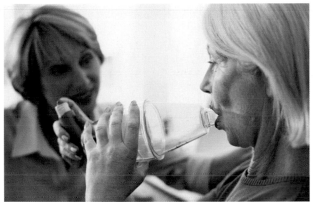

Using an inhaler with a spacer
A spacer fits on the mouthpiece of an inhaler. Pressing the drug canister releases medication into the spacer; the medication is then inhaled through the mouth.

medication. A health professional will show you how to administer medication via the inhaler, but if you are in any doubt about the proper technique, ask him or her for assistance.

For most inhalers, first remove the cap and shake the inhaler. Then hold the inhaler upright close to the person's mouth and ask him to breathe out gently. Put the mouthpiece into the person's mouth and tell him to breathe in through the mouth

with a steady, deep breath. While the person is breathing in, press down on the canister to release the medication. Encourage the person to hold his breath for 10 seconds, then repeat if required.

Many people find using an inhaler by itself difficult, so inhalers are often used with a spacer or aerochamber. These are plastic devices that attach to the mouthpiece of the inhaler. After attaching the spacer or aerochamber, ask the person to breathe out gently. Place the mouthpiece of the spacer or aerochamber into the person's mouth, and tell him to seal his lips around the mouthpiece. Then press the inhaler canister to release the medication into the spacer and ask him to breathe in slowly and deeply. Encourage the person to hold his breath for 10 seconds, then repeat if necessary. This method is known as the single-breath technique and is effective for most people. However, if the person finds it difficult, ask the health professional to teach you the multi-breath technique.

After each use, wash the inhaler mouthpiece and spacer or aerochamber in warm, soapy water, rinse, and leave to dry.

■ **Using a nebulizer** A nebulizer is a machine that vaporizes liquid medication into a fine mist that is inhaled through a facemask. Nebulizers do not require any special techniques – the medication is simply inhaled during normal breathing. After use, the facemask should be washed, rinsed, and left to dry.

Oxygen therapy
If the person has a condition in which he cannot get enough oxygen by normal breathing, supplementary oxygen will be

» DEALING WITH BREATHING PROBLEMS

needed. The person's doctor will be able to decide if the person needs oxygen all the time, on and off throughout the day, or only when he is asleep. The oxygen may be given from a tank or cylinder containing compressed or liquid oxygen, or from a machine called an oxygen concentrator, which extracts oxygen from the air. The devices most commonly used to deliver oxygen are facemasks and nasal prongs. Less commonly, a tracheal catheter may be used. This is a small, flexible tube inserted into the windpipe.

A health professional will show you how to set up and operate the oxygen equipment, and how to set the rate of oxygen flow. When having oxygen therapy, the person may experience a dry mouth, throat, or nose. If so, the health professional can provide a humidifier and show you how to attach it to the oxygen delivery system. You can also use a water-based jelly to moisturize the person's nose, and a balm such as petroleum jelly for his lips. Offer mouthwashes to help with a dry mouth, and damp cloths to wipe the face.

> **IMPORTANT!**
>
> Oxygen is a fire hazard, and if you are using it in the home you should take the following safety precautions:
>
> - Keep oxygen well away from any flames or heat sources.
> - Do not smoke or let anybody else smoke while oxygen is being used.
> - Do not use flammable products while oxygen is being used.
> - Keep a fire extinguisher within easy reach.
> - Fit fire and smoke alarms in the home.
> - Keep oxygen cylinders upright.
> - Inform your local fire service that you have oxygen at home.

Also, check the person's skin where the mask or nasal prongs touch it, to make sure they are not digging in. If he uses nasal prongs, place gauze behind his ears to prevent the tubing from rubbing the skin.

Continuous positive airway pressure

Treatment with continuous positive airway pressure (CPAP) involves using a machine to blow air or oxygen into the airways, usually via a facemask. A health professional will show you how to use the CPAP equipment and will adjust the settings specifically for the person's requirement. It is

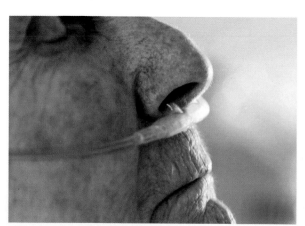

Receiving oxygen through nasal prongs

Nasal prongs are flexible plastic tubes that deliver oxygen into the nose. The prongs are connected to another pair of tubes that fit over the ears and are connected to the oxygen supply.

person's requirement. It is important that you do not alter these settings. The CPAP machine comes with a heated humidifier that warms and moistens the air. Before using the CPAP machine, you need to fill the humidifier with cooled, boiled water and connect the hoses. The CPAP equipment should be positioned close to the person so that the hoses do not restrict his movements too much.

The facemask is held in place with elasticated straps. Put the straps over the person's head, then place the mask over his mouth and nose and gently tighten the straps until the mask fits snugly and there are no leaks. Be careful not to overtighten the straps, to avoid rubbing and bruising. You should make sure you know how to remove the mask quickly, in case the person vomits.

Initially, the person may have a feeling of claustrophobia when wearing the mask, but this feeling usually wears off with continued use. He may also find it difficult to get used to air being blown into his airways. If this is a problem, consult a health professional. It may be possible to start therapy with the CPAP machine on a low setting and then gradually increase it so that the person has time to become accustomed to it. If, despite using the humidifier, the person suffers from a dry nose and mouth from CPAP, his doctor can prescribe a spray to alleviate the problem.

After each use, you should clean the mask, humidifier, and hoses of the CPAP machine with warm, soapy water, rinse well, and dry thoroughly.

Physiotherapy

In some cases, physiotherapy can help to improve breathing problems. A health professional will be able to advise if he or she thinks physiotherapy may be beneficial for the person in your care. If so, a physiotherapist will assess the person's breathing problems and suggest appropriate therapy, such as breathing exercises or chest percussion.

There are various different breathing exercises, and the ones recommended will be tailored specifically for the person in your care. They may involve special relaxation exercises to reduce the effort needed to breathe effectively or exercises to help the person control the rate and depth of his breathing by inhaling and exhaling in a slightly different way from usual. Chest percussion may be suggested if the person has difficulty coughing and clearing his chest of mucus. This involves clapping the person's chest with cupped hands to loosen the mucus. The physiotherapist will teach you how to do this correctly.

If the person has mobility problems, lack of movement may worsen breathing problems by reducing his ability to breathe deeply. In such cases, physiotherapy may help to improve mobility, which, in turn, may benefit the breathing problems.

When to get medical help

If breathing difficulty is due to an obstruction in the airway, see p.178. If breathing difficulty is accompanied by swelling of the face, mouth, or throat, and an itchy rash, it may be due to a severe allergic reaction (known as anaphylaxis); see p.187.

In other cases, you should get urgent medical help if the person's breathing difficulty is unusual (for example, not due to physical exertion) or is a new symptom. You should also get urgent medical help if any prescribed treatment for a breathing problem is ineffective, or if the breathing problem gets worse or is accompanied by other symptoms, for example a blue tinge to the lips or fingers, coughing up blood, or chest pain.

DEALING WITH VOMITING AND DIARRHOEA

Most people have experienced an occasional bout of vomiting or diarrhoea, and, although unpleasant, it is not usually a cause for concern. There are many possible causes of vomiting and/or diarrhoea. They are commonly due to an intestinal infection but may also be caused by medication, anxiety, certain medical conditions, or sometimes simply by eating or drinking too much. Whatever the cause, the advice given here will help you to deal with the problem safely and effectively.

Dealing with vomiting

If the person you are caring for is vomiting, help him into a position where he will not inhale or choke on the vomit – either sitting upright with his head tilted forwards,or lying on his side. Check that the room is cool and well ventilated, and make sure there is always a clean vomit bowl to hand. Remove used bowls immediately and clean them thoroughly; wash and dry your hands afterwards. Offer the person mouthwash or water to rinse out his mouth and a damp cloth to wipe his face. It is also vital to ensure that the person does not become dehydrated (opposite). After the person has recovered from an episode of vomiting, it is advisable to give him bland, easily digestible food for the next few meals.

If the person takes prescribed medication, particularly oral medication, vomiting may have prevented proper absorption of the medication. You should therefore consult the person's doctor about when to give the next dose. In some cases, the doctor may also suggest adjustments to the medication (see panel, right).

■ **When to get medical help** Seek urgent medical help if the person is vomiting persistently, if there is blood in the vomit, if you suspect the person has inhaled vomit, or if there are other symptoms in addition to the vomiting.

Dealing with diarrhoea

Diarrhoea is often accompanied by a frequent need to defecate and difficulty in controlling bowel movements, or even complete loss of bowel control. If the person is suffering from diarrhoea, you should therefore ensure he has close and easy access to the toilet. You should also make sure there is a good supply of items for personal hygiene, odour-eliminating products, and, if necessary, incontinence pads. If the person's clothes or bedding become soiled, they should be replaced and the soiled items washed immediately. You should also make sure that you wash your own hands thoroughly and frequently.

Diarrhoea causes a rapid loss of body fluids, so you should encourage the person to drink plenty of clear fluids

---

ADJUSTING MEDICATION

If the person you are caring for takes medication and is vomiting or has diarrhoea, absorption of the medication may be reduced and you should consult the person's doctor.

■ The doctor will be able to advise about the dosage regimen and may also suggest giving medication by a different route – for example, by injection or rectal suppository rather than by mouth.

■ If the vomiting and/or diarrhoea are due to the medication itself, the doctor may be able to prescribe an alternative.

■ In some cases, the doctor may be able to prescribe medication that helps prevent diarrhoea and/or vomiting.

to prevent dehydration (see below). Until the diarrhoea has subsided, you should give the person a soft, bland diet, and avoid giving foods that are high in fibre or fat.

Frequent bowel movements may cause sore skin in the rectal area. If so, bathe the area in warm water, pat dry with a soft, clean towel, and apply barrier or haemorrhoid cream to help relieve any pain.

Do not give the person any over-the-counter antidiarrhoea medications without first checking with the person's doctor or other health professional, because the antidiarrhoea medications may interact with other medications the person is taking. If the diarrhoea is caused by an intestinal infection, antidiarrhoea medications may even prolong the problem. Diarrhoea can sometimes result in inadequate absorption of medications. If the person takes prescribed medication, you should consult the doctor for advice.

■ **When to get medical help** Seek prompt medical advice if there is blood in the diarrhoea, or if the diarrhoea lasts for more than 48 hours or is accompanied by other symptoms.

Dealing with dehydration

Dehydration is a potentially serious problem for somebody suffering from vomiting or diarrhoea. It is therefore essential to take measures to prevent it, and also to be aware of the signs so that you can take corrective measures promptly.

The best way to prevent the person from becoming dehydrated is by making sure he drinks plenty of water (or other clear fluids) frequently throughout the day. To make water more palatable, try adding a slice of lemon or orange. If the person has a fever, he will have lost electrolytes,

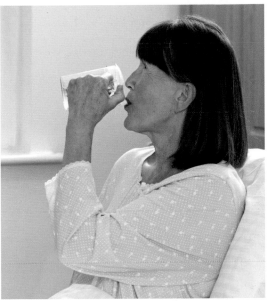

Helping a person to drink
You may find it easier to give fluids using a special drinking cup or, if this is impractical, a syringe to gently squirt liquid into the mouth.

such as salt. Giving an over-the-counter oral rehydration solution will help to replace these.

Early signs of dehydration include thirst, a dry mouth, reduced urine output, and dark-coloured urine. The skin also becomes less elastic. You can test this by gently squeezing the skin of the person's forearm between your thumb and index finger; if he is well hydrated, his skin will spring back straight away, whereas it will take a few seconds to do so if he is dehydrated. If the person is only slightly dehydrated, increasing his fluid intake will usually correct the problem.

■ **When to get medical help** You should get urgent medical help if the person is showing signs of severe dehydration. Such signs include an increased breathing rate, increased heart rate, dizziness, irritability, confusion, lethargy, and, in extremely severe cases, unconsciousness.

9

FIRST AID EMERGENCIES

WHAT TO DO IN AN EMERGENCY

When a person is injured it is essential that you stay calm and follow a clear plan of action. First and foremost, consider your own safety, and only approach the person if you know it's safe to do so. If it's not safe, call the emergency services and keep your distance. Monitor the person from where you are standing and don't approach her even if the condition appears to worsen.

Setting priorities

If a person has fallen, leave her where she is unless her life is in danger. Assess her condition and/or injuries and only move her if you are certain that doing so will not exacerbate any injury.

Deal with life-threatening injuries first. If, for example, a person is unconscious, it is important to establish that she is breathing normally (opposite) before you treat any other injury she may have. If she is conscious and breathing, check for injuries and treat any obvious bleeding to prevent shock (p.181). Assess the level of consciousness: is she alert and awake, or does she only respond to voice or pain?

Then, carry out a more detailed examination of the person. Make her comfortable and listen to what she has to say. If she fell, she may tell you, for example, that she has hurt her arm or leg. However, if you saw her fall you may have

CALLING FOR HELP

If a person has a minor injury, you may be able to treat it at home. If you are in any doubt, seek medical advice by calling the person's GP surgery. The receptionist will either put you in contact with a nurse or the doctor, depending on the condition. If a person needs hospital treatment but can walk, and her condition is unlikely to deteriorate, you can take her by car. Call 999 for an ambulance if a person is seriously ill or injured as she will need specialist help on the journey.

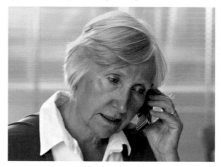

Giving information
Tell the operator as much as you can about the incident and the person. Mention any underlying conditions the person suffers from.

noticed that she banged her head as well. If necessary carry out a quick head-to-toe check, comparing the injured side of the body with the uninjured side. Write down anything you notice as it may be of use to the paramedic or doctor later.

FIRST AID KITS

Even if you have a medical kit at home, it is worth having a separate first aid kit. You can buy a ready-made one or make up your own. First aid equipment should be kept in a clean water-tight container. It is worth having two – one at home and another one in the car in case of an incident while you are out. Keep a list in each box of any medication that the person you are caring for has to take.

Useful items to keep
- Dressings and bandages – keep a variety of adhesive dressings, sterile pads, roller bandages, and a triangular bandage.

- Antiseptic wipes, gauze swabs for cleaning a wound, and disposable gloves.

- Scissors, safety pins, adhesive tape, tweezers, instant cold pack, torch, note pad, and pencil.

UNCONSCIOUSNESS

If a person collapses apparently unconscious, act quickly. Check his breathing as there is a risk that it could stop, especially if he is lying on his back as his tongue can fall back, blocking the air passages to the lungs. Call for emergency help as quickly as possible – ideally get someone else to do this – as the faster the person receives specialist help, the greater the chances of survival.

1 Gently shake the person's shoulders. Speaking clearly, call his name or ask him to open his eyes, then watch for a response; if there is no response he is unconscious.

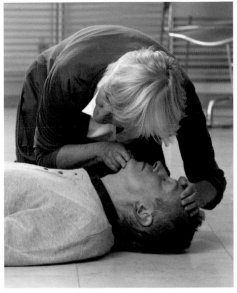

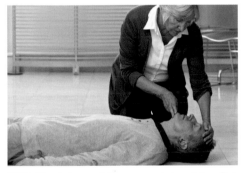

2 Check to see if the person is breathing. Put one hand on his forehead and gently tilt his head back. Then put two fingers of your other hand on the tip of the chin and lift it.

3 With the head in this position the tongue can't fall back and block the airway. Put your ear as close as possible to the person's nose and mouth. Listen and feel for breaths and at the same time, look along his chest watching for movement.

4 If the person is breathing, place him in the recovery position, see below, and call an ambulance. If he is not breathing, call an amublance, then begin CPR (cardiopulmonary resuscitation), pp.176–177.

RECOVERY POSITION

Place an unconscious person who is breathing in this recovery position to allow fluid to drain from his mouth and keep his airways open. Place him on his side with the lower leg straight and the upper leg bent at the knee and hip to prevent him rolling forward. Tilt his head back slightly and bend his upper arm, placing his hand under his chin to support it.

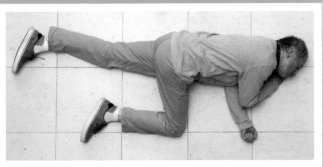

CPR

If a collapsed person is not breathing, oxygen will not reach vital organs such as the brain, and his heartbeat will eventually stop (cardiac arrest). Cardiopulmonary resuscitation, or CPR – a combination of chest compressions and rescue breaths – can help maintain an oxygen supply to the body. You start with chest compressions to restore blood circulation because when breathing stops the oxygen level in the blood remains the same initially. After a few minutes oxygen levels drop, then you need to start rescue breaths.

> **IMPORTANT!**
>
> - If you are on your own, call 999 for an ambulance before you begin.
>
> - Do not press on the ribs or the lower part of the breastbone when giving compressions.
>
> - If you have help when giving CPR, swap over every 1–2 minutes (without interrupting a sequence of compressions).

AEDs can save lives

The most common cause of cardiac arrest is ventricular fibrillation, or an abnormal heart rhythm. Delivering a controlled shock as soon as possible from a machine called an automated external defibrillator (AED) can correct this.

Many public places are equipped with AEDs and they are carried by the emergency services. When you ask someone to call an ambulance for a person who is not breathing, tell him or her to ask for an AED. Start CPR (see below), then use the machine as soon as it arrives (see opposite).

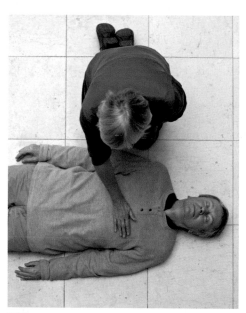

1 Make sure the person is lying on his back on a firm surface. Kneel beside him level with his chest, and place one hand on the centre of his chest.

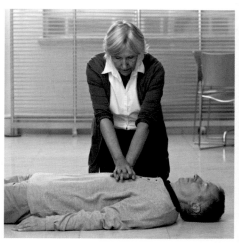

2 Place your other hand on top of the first hand. Interlock your fingers but keep them raised off the chest. Lean directly over the person's chest, straighten your arms, and press down on the breastbone to depress it 5–6cm (2–2½in). Release the pressure, but don't move your hands – let the chest come back up. Repeat to give 30 chest compressions at a rate of about 100 to 120 per minute.

HOW TO USE AN AED

These machines can be used without any prior training. The AED will give you a series of visual or verbal prompts to follow. If the person recovers at any point, leave the pads in position and wait for the ambulance to arrive.

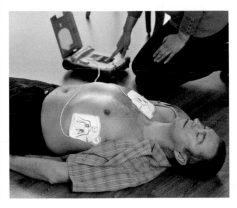

1 Switch on the machine. Take out the pads and position them on the person's chest and side as shown on the pack.

2 Make sure no-one is touching the person. The AED will analyse him, and visual or aural instructions then indicate whether or not a shock is advised.

3 If a shock is advised, make sure everyone stands clear, then press the shock button; the person may appear to "jump". You will then be told to continue CPR for 2 minutes, when it will re-analyse the person.

4 If no shock is advised, you will be told to continue CPR for 2 minutes, when it will re-analyse the person.

Positioning the pads
Remove the adhesive backing and place one pad on the upper right side of the person's chest and the other on his left side, near his armpit.

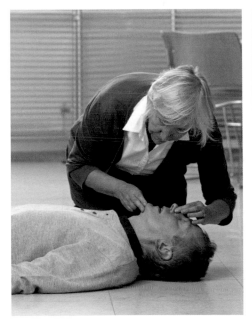

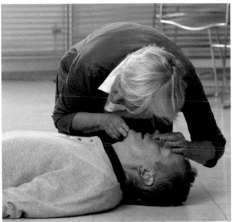

4 Remove your mouth, but keep the nostrils closed and maintain the chin lift. Look along the person's chest to watch it fall. Repeat to give a second breath. If the chest didn't rise, adjust the head and try again. Don't try more than twice.

3 Move towards the person's head and open the airway; put one hand on his forehead and pinch his nostrils shut, and put two fingers of the other hand on the tip of the chin to lift it. Take a breath, seal your lips around the person's mouth, and blow into it until his chest rises.

5 Repeat compressions followed by rescue breaths at a rate of 30:2 until emergency help arrives, the person shows signs of regaining consciousness (for example, coughing, opening his eyes, speaking, *and* moving purposefully), or you are too exhausted to continue.

CHOKING

If food "goes down the wrong way" it can become stuck in the throat, which blocks the airway and causes muscle spasm. If the blockage is mild, the person may be able to cough it clear; if it is severe, breathing will stop and you must act quickly to clear it. Elderly people are more at risk from choking as they often have difficulty chewing food and may find coughing difficult.

1 If the person can talk and breathe, encourage her to cough and don't intervene. Tell her to spit out anything in her mouth, or you can help her. Pick out anything you can see.

2 If she can't speak or she stops coughing and/or breathing, use back blows to try to free the blockage. Stand beside her and help her to lean forwards. Support her upper body with one hand and, using the heel of your hand, give up to five sharp back blows between her shoulders. Stop back blows if the obstruction is cleared, and tell her to spit out the object.

3 If the airway is still blocked, try abdominal thrusts. Help her to bend forwards, then stand behind her. Put your arms around the upper part of her abdomen – between the bottom of the breastbone and the belly button. Place one clenched fist against the person's abdomen and grasp it with your other hand. Pull sharply inwards and upwards up to five times.

4 Check the person's mouth again. If she still can't cough, speak, or breathe, repeat steps 2 and 3 up to three times.

5 If the person is still choking, call an ambulance, or ask someone to make the call for you. Continue back blows and abdominal thrusts until help arrives.

IMPORTANT!

If the person becomes unconscious at any stage, call an ambulance. Open the airway and check breathing:

- If she is breathing, place her in the recovery position.
- If she is not breathing begin CPR (pp.176–177) as this may relieve the obstruction.

SYMPTOMS AND SIGNS

- A person will suddenly start coughing or gasping for breath. Ask her if she is choking.
- If the airway is partially blocked, she will be able to talk, cough, and breathe.
- If person cannot talk, cough, or breathe, the airway is completely blocked.

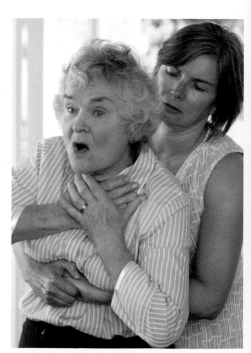

SEVERE CHEST PAIN

Sudden and very severe chest pain is often a symptom of a heart attack. It is normally caused by an obstruction in the arteries that supply blood to the heart muscle, usually a blood clot. Angina can occur when the blood supply is restricted, see below. The outcome of a heart attack will depend on how much muscle is affected and how quickly the person receives medical treatment. He is likely to be very frightened by the pain so it is important to reassure him and stay calm.

SYMPTOMS AND SIGNS

- Persistent, vice-like pain that spreads to the jaw and down one or both arms and does not go away if the person rests.
- Feeling of discomfort in the abdomen similar to indigestion.
- Person will be breathless and may be gasping for air.
- Possible pale, greyish skin that feels clammy or sweaty – lips may be blue.
- Person may feel faint and dizzy and may collapse without warning.
- Pulse can be rapid, weak, and irregular
- Possible loss of consciouness.

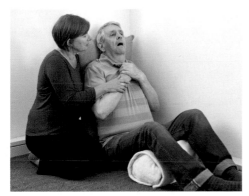

1 Make the person as comfortable possible in a half-sitting position with his head, shoulders, and back supported and his knees bent. This will ease the pain and any strain on his heart.

2 Call an ambulance, or get someone to make the call for you. Tell the operator that the person may have had a heart attack.

3 Unless you know he is allergic to aspirin, give him a full-dose (300mg) tablet to limit the extent of the muscle damage. Tell him to chew it slowly , rather than taking it with water. If he has angina medication (a pump spray or tablets), help him to take that too.

4 Monitor the person's level of response, breathing, and pulse, while you wait for the ambulance. Make a note of any changes, and tell the paramedics when they arrive.

ANGINA

This is a condition caused by narrowing of the arteries that supply the heart muscle. As a result they cannot supply the muscle with enough blood to meet its needs during exertion. This causes chest pain, which forces the person to rest and the pain normally eases. Anyone diagnosed with angina will be given medication for use in an attack.

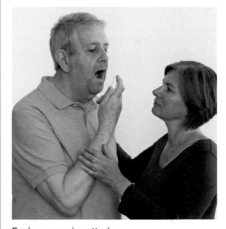

Easing an angina attack
Help the person to sit down and rest and let him take his medication. The pain should ease within a few minutes of taking it.

BLEEDING

Loss of blood from a wound can be dramatic and frightening for the person. It is vital that it is controlled as quickly as possible to prevent too much blood being lost from the circulatory system (see Shock, opposite). Some elderly people have also been prescribed blood-thinning medication (anticoagulants), so will bleed profusely after a minor injury. If the bleeding is severe, don't give the person anything to eat or drink as she may need surgery.

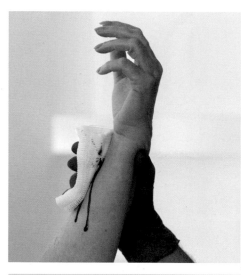

1 Apply pressure directly over the injured area straight away. Ideally, put a sterile or clean pad over the wound first, or use your hand.

2 Raise the injured area above the level of the person's heart; this slows down the blood flow to the injury. Help her to sit down.

3 Place a pad on the wound if you have not already done so, then tie a bandage around it. The bandage should be firm enough to help maintain the pressure, but not so tight that it restricts circulation to the limb beyond the injury.

4 Help the person to support the injured area in a raised position. Seek medical advice. If the bleeding is severe, call an ambulance.

BLEEDING AT SPECIAL SITES

SITE OF BLEEDING	WHAT TO DO
Nosebleed	Help her to sit down and tell her to lean her head forward and pinch the soft part of her nose: she should spit out any blood in her mouth. Release pressure after 10 minutes and, if bleeding continues, reapply.
Burst varicose vein	Veins in the legs have one-way valves to ensure blood flow to the heart. If they fail, blood can "pool" in the veins and severe bleeding can result from a minor knock. Lay the person down and raise the leg immediately to slow blood flow to the area, then apply direct pressure.
Scalp wound	The scalp has many blood vessels, so a small knock can cause profuse bleeding. Apply direct pressure over a pad, then sit the person on the floor – don't lie her down. Secure the pad with a bandage.
Bleeding from mouth	If the lips are bleeding, cover wound with a pad and squeeze it. Place a gauze pad in a bleeding tooth socket and tell the person to bite on it.

SHOCK

Medical shock is a life-threatening condition that will develop if large amounts of fluid are lost from the body, for example as a result of bleeding or burns. If there isn't enough body fluid, the circulatory system fails and can't provide the vital organs such as the heart and brain with oxygen-rich blood. Shock can be exacerbated by fear so it is important to reassure the person and make her as comfortable as possible while you wait for help.

SYMPTOMS AND SIGNS

The following symptoms and signs will gradually worsen.

- Rapid pulse at first, which gradually weakens. When half the circulating blood is lost, you won't feel a pulse at the wrist.

- Cold, clammy skin and sweating. As the shock develops, the skin will become grey-blue – this will be most obvious on the ears, lips, inside the mouth, and fingertips. If you press a fingernail, the normal pink colour will not return quickly.

- Weakness and dizziness, with nausea and possible vomiting.

- The person will become very thirsty.

- As oxygen to the brain reduces, the person will become aggressive and restless. She will yawn and gasp for air.

- Unconsciousness – the heart may stop altogether.

IMPORTANT!

- Never give a person with suspected shock a hot-water bottle or electric blanket to keep her warm as it draws blood to the skin and away from the vital organs of the body.

- Do not give the person anything to eat or drink as she may need an anaesthetic in hospital later.

- If she is thirsty, moisten her lips with water.

- Any bleeding from body openings such as ear, mouth, or nose may be a sign of internal bleeding.

1 Treat any obvious cause of injury – for example, apply direct pressure to control severe bleeding (see opposite) or cool a burn p.185).

2 Reassure the person and help her to lie down, if necessary on a blanket to protect her from a cold floor. Don't put anything under her head. Raise her legs as high as you can and support them, for example, resting her feet on a chair. If she has broken a bone in her leg, raise the uninjured leg only.

3 Loosen any tight clothing, especially at the neck, chest, and waist as it can restrict blood flow around the body. Cover the person with a blanket to keep her warm.

4 Call an ambulance. Check the person's level of response, breathing, and pulse, while you wait for help. Make a note of any changes, and tell the paramedics when they arrive.

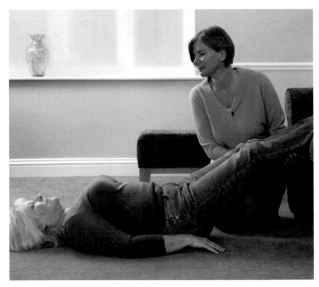

HEAD INJURY

A blow to the head is potentially serious.
Even an apparently minor bump can affect a person's level of consciousness. A blow can cause the brain to be literally "shaken" inside the skull, causing a temporary disturbance in the brain and even unconsciousness. This is known as concussion and the person may be unaware of what happened, but will recover soon afterwards. An injury can also cause bleeding within the brain, or between the brain and the skull, which causes a build-up of pressure within the skull – a compression injury. This is very serious and the symptoms may not be evident for hours or even days after the incident. There may be a scalp wound and these often bleed profusely (p.180).

SYMPTOMS AND SIGNS

- A short period of unconsciousness after a blow to the head.
- The person may not remember anything that happened just before or after the injury.

The injury needs urgent medical attention if you notice the following (signs of a compression injury):

- Headache that becomes progressively worse.
- Indented area of the skull – this indicates possible skull fracture.
- Watery, bloodstained fluid leaking from the ears, nose, or mouth, which can be a sign of skull fracture.
- Person becomes increasingly drowsy or confused.
- Unexplained vomiting.
- Dizziness and/or loss of balance, even a seizure (p.186).
- Changes in breathing pattern.

IMPORTANT!

- Don't give the person anything to eat or drink; seek medical advice if the person needs to take prescription medication.
- If you are in any doubt about a person's condition after a head injury, seek medical advice.

1 If the person is fully conscious, help her to sit down in a comfortable chair, or sit her up if she has fallen over. She is safer on the floor as she cannot fall if she feels unwell. If she is not fully conscious, call an ambulance.

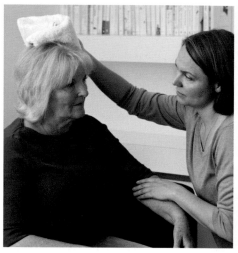

2 Hold a cold pack such as a bag of frozen peas or ice wrapped in a towel against the injury for up to 10 minutes to minimize swelling.

3 Stay with the person and encourage her to rest. If she does not recover completely within 30 minutes, her symptoms change, or her level of consciousness begins to deteriorate, seek medical advice.

4 If the person begins to appear drowsy or confused, help her to lie down, and call an ambulance. Monitor her level of consciousness, pulse, and breathing while you are waiting. Make a note of any changes.

SUSPECTED STROKE

Sometimes called a brain attack, a stroke occurs when the blood supply to the brain is cut off by a blockage in one of the arteries, or it can follow bleeding into the brain from a damaged blood vessel. It is important to get the person to hospital as soon as possible as medication can minimize the extent of the damage and help recovery. Use the FAST (Face-Arms-Speech-Time) test to confirm whether or not a person has suffered a stroke.

SYMPTOMS AND SIGNS

- Facial weakness noticeable on one side of the face.
- Arm (and/or leg) weakness down one side of his body. He may even collapse suddenly.
- Difficulty speaking.
- Difficulty swallowing.
- Person may complain of sudden weakness, or numbness, which can result in paralysis along one side of his body.
- Problems with balance and coordination.
- Person is unusually confused and has difficulty understanding what you are saying.
- Sudden, severe headache.
- Possible blurred vision or even loss of sight.
- If the stroke is caused by a burst blood vessel there will be signs of compression injury (see opposite).

MINISTROKE

If someone has any of the above symptoms, but they only last a few minutes, then he recovers, he may have had a ministroke, or transient ischaemic attack (TIA). This occurs when the blood supply is temporarily interrupted, and the symptoms normally improve quickly and disappear completely within 24 hours. A ministroke is still a medical emergency as it can be a sign that a major stroke will occur in the near future. The person should seek medical advice or go to the accident and emergency department.

1 Check for FACIAL weakness. Look at the person's face and ask him to smile. If he has had a stroke he may only be able to smile on one side, and the eye and mouth on the affected side may droop.

2 Check for ARM weakness. Ask the person to lift his arms. If he has had a stroke he may only be able to lift one arm.

3 Do you notice any SPEECH difficulty? Talk to him. Speech can be impaired after a stroke, or he may not be able to understand you.

4 It's TIME to call an ambulance if the person fails any of these tests.

BONE, JOINT, & MUSCLE INJURIES

It is very difficult to differentiate between a broken bone and a joint injury without an X-ray. If in doubt, treat every injury as a break. The aim of treatment is to prevent movement in the injured area damaging the nerves and body tissue around the injury. Elderly people can easily break a bone if they fall. Common injuries are broken "hip" (top of the thighbone), and fractured wrist, which results from falling onto an outstretched hand.

- Don't give her anything to eat or drink as she may need an anaesthetic in hospital.
- Never try to straighten an injured limb.
- Control bleeding by covering wound with a clean pad and apply pressure *around* it.

SYMPTOMS AND SIGNS

- Pain and difficulty moving the injured area.
- Swelling and later bruising around the site of the injury.
- Obvious deformity if you compare the injured limb to the uninjured one. If a leg is broken, one leg may appear shorter than the other.
- Person may tell you that she can feel bone ends moving.
- There may be a wound above the break.
- Possible signs of shock (p.181) if a large bone, such as the thighbone, is injured as this can cause internal bleeding.

1 Encourage the person to support the injury by hand, or do it for her. Make her comfortable – on the floor if she can't get up.

2 Immobilize the injury to prevent damage to surrounding tissue, using rolled towels, blankets, or pillows. If it's a sprain or strain place a cold pack against it to minimize swelling.

3 If an arm is injured and the person is mobile, you can drive her to hospital. For any other injury call an ambulance as she may need to be transported on a stretcher.

4 Reassure the person and monitor her condition while you wait for help.

SPECIAL SITES OF INJURY

INJURY	WHAT TO DO
Wrist and hand	Wrap a towel around the injury and help the person support the injured arm so that her hand is higher than her elbow.
Elbow	If the elbow can be bent, treat as above. If she can't bend the arm, lay it across her lap and support with cushions.
Leg	Leave the person in the position found. Place rolled-up towels or blankets along each side of the injured leg to prevent movement.
Pelvis	Place rolled blankets along either side of both legs. Ask her to bend her legs slightly if she can, then slide a cushion under her knees.
Knee	Help the person lie down and support the knee in a bent postion with a few cushions. Wrap soft padding around it.

BURNS

A burn can damage the surface of the skin, just the top layer, or all the layers (see panel, below) and some injuries have areas of all three. It is essential to cool a burn as quickly as possible to stop the burning process. This type of injury is potentially serious as it can allow fluid to be lost from the circulatory system, which can result in shock (p.181). In addition, as burns can affect a large area of skin, there is a high risk of infection.

TYPES OF BURN

- *Superficial burns* affect the surface of the skin. The skin will be red and swollen.

- *Partial-thickness burns* affect the top layer of skin. As the skin is broken, fluid (plasma) can escape. These burns are painful, skin will be red and raw, and blisters may form.

- *Deep burns* damage all the layers of skin. As nerves may be affected they can be pain-free. The blood vessels and muscle beneath the skin may also be damaged.

IMPORTANT!

- Never break blisters resulting from a burn.

- Don't put any creams, ointments, or fats on a burn.

- Never put an adhesive dressing over a burn; the injured area may extend further than you think and removing the dressing may tear the damaged skin.

- Don't use specialized dressings, gels, or sprays unless specifically advised to by the medical team.

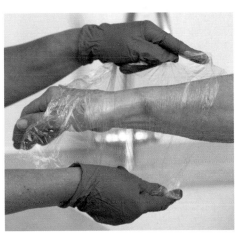

1 Cool the injured area as quickly as possible to stop the burning and minimize swelling. Hold the area under cold running water for about 10 minutes, or until it stops hurting. Don't overcool the person. If there's no water available you can use milk or canned drinks.

2 While you are cooling the area, remove any clothing or jewellery before it starts to swell. Cut the clothing if necessary, but don't remove anything that is stuck to the burn.

3 Raise and support the injury. Cover the burn with a length of plastic kitchen film; don't wrap it around a limb. You can cover a hand or foot with a clean plastic bag. If neither is available, use a clean cotton or linen cloth.

4 Seek medical advice for any burn larger than 2.5cm (1in). Call an ambulance for: partial-thickness burns larger than the palm of the person's hand; a burn that extends all the way around a limb, even if superficial; any full-thickness burn; burns affecting the mouth.

5 If the burn is severe, treat for shock (p.181) while waiting for help to arrive.

BRUISING

A fall or knock that does not break the skin can result in bleeding into the tissues. Bruising can develop quickly or may not be evident for some hours after the injury. It will be more severe if a person is taking anticoagulants.

1 Help the person to sit down, or make her comfortable on the floor if she has fallen. Raise the injury above the level of her heart to reduce blood flow to the area.

2 Cool the injury and minimize swelling by placing a bag of ice or pack of frozen peas wrapped in a towel against the injury for up to 10 minutes; don't let the area become too cold.

IMPORTANT!

- If a person develops bruises and there was no obvious cause, seek medical advice.
- If you suspect serious injury, call an ambulance.

3 If the pain and/or swelling is severe, wrap soft padding around the injury for extra support. Seek medical advice.

SEIZURES

A seizure is caused by a disturbance in the electrical activity within the brain. Commonly caused by epilepsy, seizures can also occur in a person suffering from a disease that affects the brain or after a head injury.

1 If a person starts to have a seizure, clear a space around her. Don't try to prevent her from falling or restrain her in any way as you could be injured. Place soft padding around her or against furniture. Put rolled towels or cushions around her head for further protection.

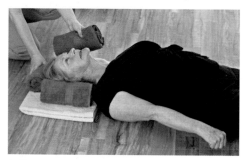

2 When the convulsive movements stop, she may be very sleepy. Put her in the recovery position (p.175).

3 Make a note of how long the convulsions lasted. Monitor her condition as she recovers. If she is known to suffer from seizures, seek medical advice. If she has never had a seizure, call an ambulance.

IMPORTANT!

Call an ambulance if:
- A seizure lasts for more than 10 minutes, or is followed straight away by another one.
- She is unconscious for over 10 minutes after the seizure.

STAGES OF SEIZURE

Seizures normally follow a pattern:

- Person collapses suddenly.
- She becomes rigid and may arch her back.
- Jerky, or convulsive, movements begin. She may also lose control of bowel or bladder.
- Breathing may be difficult as she clenches her jaw – lips may appear blue or grey. There may be blood around her mouth if she has bitten her lip or tongue.
- Muscles relax and breathing is normal.
- Person regains consciousness, but may be very drowsy and fall into a deep sleep. When she wakes she may not remember anything.

INSECT STING

Most insect stings are more painful than dangerous. However, they can cause a serious allergic reaction in a person who is susceptible. A sting in the mouth can result in severe swelling and/or a blocked airway so should be treated as an emergency.

SYMPTOMS AND SIGNS

- Redness at the site of injury; a bee's sting may still be in the skin.

- Swelling around the site of the sting(s).

- Possible itchy rash if a mild allergic reaction develops.

1 Sit the person down. If you can see the sting, slide a credit card underneath it and scrape it off. Don't try to pull it out with your fingers as you may squeeze poison into the area.

2 Place a bag of ice or frozen peas wrapped in a towel against the area to reduce swelling. Raise the injured area to help to minimize the swelling. If the sting is in the mouth give the person an ice cube to suck.

3 Reassure the person. Check her regularly, watching especially for signs of severe allergic reaction (below). If she is known to be affected by insect stings, seek medical advice. If the sting is in the mouth, call an ambulance.

SEVERE ALLERGIC REACTION

This is a life-threatening condition, also called anaphylactic shock, that affects the entire body within minutes of contact with a trigger. This is an emergency. People known to have serious allergies often carry a pack containing a syringe of adrenaline.

SYMPTOMS AND SIGNS

- Red itchy rash – skin will look flushed – often affecting the entire body.

- Swelling around the face and mouth.

- Person finds breathing very difficult, her chest may feel tight, or she may be wheezing and gasping for air.

- Tongue and throat may be swollen, and her eyes will look puffy.

- She will find it difficult to swallow – this gradually worsens.

- Person may be frightened and agitated.

- Symptoms and signs of shock (p.181), leading to loss of consciousness.

1 Call an ambulance and tell the operator that the person is having an allergic reaction.

2 If the person has an adrenaline syringe help her to administer it. Remove the safety cap and, gripping the syringe with your fist, place the tip against the thigh (through the clothing)and press hard.

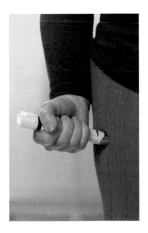

3 Help the person into the most comfortable breathing position. Monitor the person's breathing, pulse, and level of consciousness while you wait for the ambulance. If she becomes pale and pulse is weak, lie her down and raise her legs.

EFFECTS OF COLD

Anyone who is immobile or frail is more susceptible to the effects of cold, and in particular hypothermia, a condition that develops when the core body temperature falls below 35°C (95°F). When this happens the body shuts down the blood supply to the extremities to keep the vital organs supplied with blood. If not reversed, hypothermia can be fatal. Elderly people often lose their sensitivity to the cold so may not be aware of a drop in body temperature. It is important that a person suffering from hypothermia is rewarmed gradually as rapid warming can trigger a stroke or a heart attack.

IMPORTANT!

- Never put an elderly person in a bath to warm her as it can send too much blood to the heart too quickly.
- Hypothermia can mask the symptoms of a heart attack (p.179) or stroke (p.183).
- Don't rub the skin to warm her.
- Don't give the person alcohol; it dilates the blood vessels.

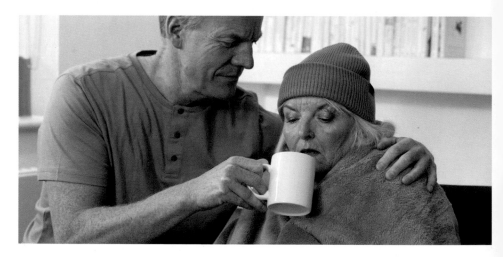

SYMPTOMS AND SIGNS

- Skin will feel cold and dry, and she will be very pale.
- Person may be shivering. This stops in the later stage.
- Lack of energy. Person will become disorientated and irrational.
- Breathing becomes slow and shallow and eventually stops.
- Pulse becomes slow, weak, and irregular if hypothermia is not reversed.
- Possible unconsciousness. If this develops begin CPR (p.176).

1 Prevent the person losing more heat. If the room is cold, start to warm it up, or help the person to move to a warmer room. Wrap her in several layers of clothes and/or blankets; warm air will be trapped between the layers. Put a hat on her head. Don't give her a hot-water bottle or electric blanket as it draws blood to the skin and away from vital organs

2 If the person is fully conscious, give her a warm drink – hold it for her if she's shivering. Give her some high-energy food such as chocolate.

3 Call an ambulance. Monitor her breathing and pulse while you are waiting for help; make a note of any change.

HEAT-RELATED ILLNESS

As people age their bodies are less able to adapt to high temperatures. Certain medical conditions, such as heart failure, diabetes, and chronic obstructive pulmonary disease, increase the risk of overheating. Some medications can also cause dehydration or affect the ability of the heart, blood vessels, or sweat glands to respond to the heat. Heat exhaustion develops when a person sweats a lot and becomes dehydrated. If untreated, a more serious condition called heatstroke develops when the temperature regulation system fails altogether.

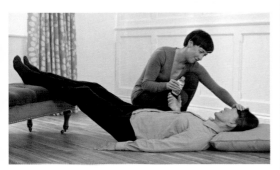

1 Move the person into a cooler room, ideally air-conditioned. Help her to lie down and rest. Raise her legs slightly.

2 Give her plenty to drink – either water or, better still, water with rehydration salts, or even isotonic drinks. Dampen a flannel with cold water and use it to cool her skin. Help her to change into lighter cotton clothing if possible.

HEATSTROKE

This is a life-threatening condition that can develop in hot weather if the body temperature rises to about 40°C (104°F) – it can develop at lower temperatures if the environment is humid. In very hot weather make sure the person is wearing light cotton clothing and stays in the shade, or in a cool room and has plenty of water to drink. If heatstroke develops:

- Call an ambulance.
- Move the person into a cool room and remove as much of her clothing as possible.
- Help her to sit down. Soak a large sheet in water and wrap it around her body to cool her. Keep the sheet damp.
- Fan her face to cool her, and open the window. Stop cooling when her body temperature falls below 37.5°C (99.5°F), and wrap her in a dry sheet.
- Monitor her condition while you are waiting for the emergency services. Re-check her body temperature every 10 minutes or so and repeat the cooling if it starts to rise.

3 Monitor the person's condition over the next couple of hours. Seek medical advice even if she appears to be recovering. If she deteriorates and/or her temperature continues to rise, call an ambulance.

SYMPTOMS AND SIGNS

Heat Exhaustion
- Person may say she feels very hot but her skin will be pale and feel cold and clammy.
- Breathing and pulse will be rapid but weak.
- She may have a headache and feel light-headed and/or faint.
- She may feel sick, and could even vomit, which worsens the dehydration.
- She may suffer muscle cramps because of the dehydration, especially in the legs.

Heatstroke
- Body temperature will be 40°C (104°F) or higher.
- Skin will appear hot, flushed, and dry.
- Pulse will be strong and "bounding".
- Person may complain of severe headache.
- Breathing may be rapid but shallow.
- Person will be confused, and her level of consciousness will deteriorate rapidly.

10

END OF LIFE CARE

■ PREPARING FOR THE END ■ IMPORTANCE OF COMMUNICATION
■ END OF LIFE DECISIONS ■ CARE OF THE DYING PERSON
■ PRACTICALITIES AFTER DEATH ■ BEREAVEMENT

PREPARING FOR THE END

There may be a time when it becomes clear that the person you are caring for may not have long to live, for example if she has been diagnosed with a terminal illness. With this realization you will naturally be distressed and have strong feelings of impending loss, yet looking after a dying person can bring great closeness between you both. The most important factor in looking after her is to help her live as well as possible in the time she has left.

How you feel

As the carer, you are likely to feel a great sense of responsibility and may be anxious over how you will deal with the emotional and practical side to your care, as well as to the emotional response of the person and her family. There are many levels of support available to help and advise you throughout the process, so you do not need to feel alone.

Getting professional support

A range of health professionals will provide support and care to the person. During this time, complex decisions must constantly be made, and it is important that you have the right information to hand, both for discussions with medical professionals as well as with the person you are caring for.

While it is hard for a doctor to give an accurate timing about the course of any illness, there may be symptoms that make it apparent when the illness is entering its final stages. The person's doctor will then consider her future medical and personal needs and develop a care plan in conjunction with the district nurse and the family.

District nurses work very closely with the doctor. They can offer day-to-day help, for example if injections or dressings are needed, and they will also coordinate and help plan her care. When discussing a care plan with you, the district nurse will suggest whether overnight or daytime nursing visits would be most suitable, as well as how frequently those visits should take place. The district nurse will decide whether to request the services of any other specialist nurse (p.13), such as the Macmillan nurses who specialize in care of

Gaining understanding

A person with a terminal illness will meet regularly with a health professional and be helped to gain understanding of her condition.

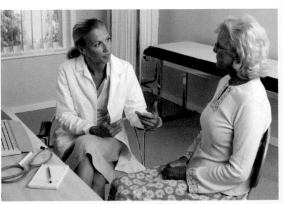

cancer patients. If the doctor and district nurse feel it is appropriate, the person you are caring for may be referred to the palliative care service.

What is palliative care?

Palliative care concentrates on relieving the uncomfortable or distressing symptoms that may be experienced by someone with a terminal illness. It treats dying as a normal process and does not aim to shorten or lengthen a person's life.

Palliative care is a free service in the UK and can be delivered through the NHS or through a charity. This type of care can be enlisted whether the person you are caring for is living in her own home, in a care home, in a hospital, or in a hospice.

■ **Assessing needs** If the person has been referred to palliative care, a nurse will do a home visit to assess her situation. The nurse will ask her (if this is possible) and you, the carer, questions about her level of activity, her appetite, whether she is suffering from any symptoms, such as nausea, depression, anxiety, or drowsiness, and what her sense of general wellbeing is like. She will be helped to express her fears of dying, whether she has worries about the family or any responsibilities she is carrying, as well as whether she is fearful of her imminent loss of independence and perhaps even the impending loss of her role in the family. The assessment will also address the needs of the carer, and the nurse will ask how you feel you are coping with the emotional and physical strain of looking after a dying person.

■ **Team approach** Palliative care utilizes many different professionals in the care of a dying person. These may be doctors, nurses, pharmacists, complementary therapists, religious leaders, social workers, psychologists, dieticians, and other allied health professionals. They all work together, and with you, to help create

a plan of care that focuses specifically on the person's individual needs and wishes.

■ **What can palliative care do?** The palliative care team offer a support system that will help the person you are caring for to live as actively and as comfortably as possible, as well as support her family and you, as her carer. Palliative care integrates all the physical, emotional, spiritual, and financial needs that arise in advanced illness and disease.

Palliative nursing care especially focuses on relieving pain and discomfort, any other side effects that the disease may be causing her in its final stages, such as shortness of breath, and any emotional distress or anxieties that she may be experiencing. Specific medicines can be offered to relieve physical symptoms; they won't cure the underlying disease but can give a quality of life back to her.

Palliative care will also offer support to you, both in terms of advice as well as practical support. If you are finding it difficult to deal with the constant demands placed on you, the palliative care team may be able to arrange extra care to enable you to have valuable time for yourself.

CARE IN A HOSPICE

Hospices specialize in care of the terminally ill, providing physical and emotional support for the person and her family, before and after death. Hospice care covers many areas:

■ Focuses on the importance of pain relief.

■ Care is not just limited to the final stages of an illness, but also helps a person live and cope with having a terminal illness.

■ Care in a hospice can be used on a short-term basis by a patient for respite care.

■ Provides physical, spiritual, social psychological, and emotional support.

■ If the person asks to be able to die at home, support from the hospice nurses will continue in the person's home.

IMPORTANCE OF COMMUNICATION

There are many people to consider when someone is dying, and as the carer your role is likely to be central. Great sensitivity is required to ensure that everyone's feelings are taken into account, not least those of the person you are caring for.

Talking to family members

Good communication among all the close family members is very important so that everyone feels involved and informed throughout the process. Whether you are a relative of the person or a friend, you will need to work out what level of involvement each of her family members would like to take. Sensitivity and patience is needed, and by planning together early on you can help to take away some of the stress during the loved one's dying phase.

Siblings need to talk frequently and keep each other abreast of any new information and share any concerns. Any disagreement on end of life care management can lead to stress, confusion, and conflict. Try to decide from the outset who is going to take responsibility for which role; for example, who will liaise with the doctor or hospital,

speak to the social worker for advice about benefits, or act as contact for the community nursing team.

Adult children naturally feel they want to protect a dying parent by not mentioning death, and the parent remains protective until the end, not wanting to mention dying in case she frightens or distresses her children. Try to encourage open dialogue, so that everyone's opinions are heard and all decisions are noted down.

Listening

It is important that the person you are caring for is consulted over who she wants to help her make decisions for her end of life care. She will need to decide which treatments she wants, as well as under what circumstances she would want treatments to stop (p.196). For example, how does she feel about life-sustaining interventions, such as nasogastric tubes (p.59), which keep someone hydrated if she is no longer able to swallow effectively or take pain relief.

A person who is dying can go through a whole range of emotions, from anger, resentment, sadness, and depression to anxiety, worry, panic, and restlessness. Talking to a religious or spiritual advisor can be an appealing option, even if the person may not have been religiously observant previously.

Many people become withdrawn in the last few weeks, perhaps due to depression or a gradual withdrawal from the world. While it may be very upsetting to see the person appearing to give up, withdrawal is a normal aspect of the dying phase and it is important to respond appropriately while the person is still able to communicate. Listen to her carefully and acknowledge, rather than deny, her feelings.

LOOKING AFTER YOURSELF

Being a carer through the dying phase means making very hard decisions. Feeling overwhelmed is a normal reaction to your circumstances and it is important to reach out for support when you need it.

- Sharing fears and worries with a friend, a professional counsellor or bereavement counselling service, or a religious leader may help you to feel better able to cope.

- The district or specialist nurses involved with the care of the person you are looking after can offer invaluable support and advice to you as the carer. You are likely to make very close bonds with them during this final phase of the person's life.

END OF LIFE DECISIONS

Once the person knows she has a terminal illness, it is very important for her to both consider and put down in writing what she would and would not like to happen as she nears the end of her life. These preferences will be taken into account as part of a plan for her advance care (see below).

Advance care planning

By encouraging the person to make an advance care plan, you will ensure that her wishes can be respected, even if she loses the capacity to make a decision due to a deterioration in her condition. There are two specific but overlapping areas within advance care planning:

■ **Advance Statement** This is a statement of the person's preferences regarding her health and social care, for example whether she would like to be cared for at home or in a hospice (p.193). An advance statement is not legally binding but is

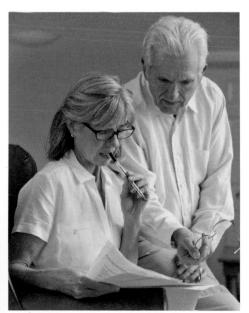

invaluable when planning care. The process of discussion can also help the person to come to terms with the fact of death and to accept a new reality. Sensitive discussion of advance care planning can strengthen coping mechanisms and enable realistic planning.

■ **Advance Decision** Also called a living will, this is a document setting out the circumstances under which the person would not want to receive life-sustaining medical treatment, for example being given cardiopulmonary resuscitation (CPR).

The person must first be assessed as being mentally competent in order for the Advance Decision to be valid, and, as long as it is accurately formulated, it can be legally binding. It can be particularly useful if the person has not appointed a health and welfare attorney under a Lasting Power of Attorney (LPA; below), as in this instance there would be no one legally able to make decisions on her behalf. However, if there is no LPA and no Advance Decision has been made in relation to a particular treatment, a doctor will make a decision for the person based on a medical assessment of her best interests.

Appointing someone to make decisions

If the person is worried that she may become incapable of making decisions for herself, she can appoint an attorney to make decisions for her, by making an LPA. This needs to be registered with the Office of the Public Guardian (p.213) before it can be used. There are two types of LPA: one for decisions about the person's health and

Planning ahead
Making plans for the future does not have to be frightening. Sitting down with a friend or relative to discuss options can be uplifting for both parties.

welfare (LPA for Health and Welfare, discussed here), the other for decisions about her property and finances (LPA for Property and Financial Affairs, p.210).

An LPA for Health and Welfare authorizes an attorney to make decisions such as when to refuse medical treatment as well as where the person should live and how she should be cared for. There is some overlap with Advance Decisions. An LPA for Health and Welfare must be made before the person loses the ability to make decisions for herself (known as "capacity"), but only comes into force once capacity is lost. A person can organize an LPA herself and there is guidance and the necessary forms on the government website (p.216). Alternatively, it can be organized through a solicitor. The attorney can be any adult, such as a friend, relative, or professional.

Cultural and spiritual needs

The person's spiritual needs may become an important component of her wellbeing precisely at the time when standard medical approaches have lost their curative or even life-sustaining efficacy. Questions about meaning and value arise naturally

throughout the dying phase and addressing them can be very comforting. When faced with death, the person may even develop a religious or spiritual belief where before she had none. Understanding her faith may give you a clearer structure for any difficult decisions that may need to be made in the future. Any rituals that need observing should be communicated to all her carers.

Contact with someone from her faith should be encouraged if it is an important aspect of the person's life, and requests to see a spiritual advisor should always be taken seriously, regardless of the person's previous attitude towards faith or religion.

QUESTIONS TO CONSIDER

There is much for the person nearing the end of her life to take in, and the following questions may help to focus her thoughts:

- What makes me happy right now?

- What is important to me?

- What role does spirituality or religion play in my life?

- Is there anything I haven't said which I now wish to say or sort out with someone?

- Are there any final things that I would like sorted before I die?

- What would I like to happen or not happen?

- Is there anyone I don't want to see or visitors I don't want to have?

- Do I have any specific wishes in the way I want to be cared for in my final days?

- Do I still want to be at home? Is it the best place for me to be cared for?

- Which medical interventions will I consent to, and which ones will I not?

- Are there any specific things I would like in my final days? For example, fresh flowers, music, my pet, or favourite foods?

- Do I have any specific religious or spiritual requests for my funeral?

- Do I want to be buried or cremated?

- What would I like to be buried in, and how would I like my funeral to be organized?

- Where should my final resting place be?

CARE OF THE DYING PERSON

Your main aim in caring for a dying person is to give her the best quality of life possible, by making her comfortable and keeping her occupied and positive. If at any time you think she is in pain or feeling panicky, mention it to the doctor or specialist nurse, who can help ease that symptom with an appropriate medicine.

As she deteriorates, her symptoms may become more pronounced, and she may have an increased need to sleep. This can make it harder for her to concentrate on, or take part in, what is going on around her.

A comfortable environment

Try to keep the person's environment as appealing as possible, for example fresh flowers will liven up a room and provide a pleasant fragrance, while some gentle music may help offer stimulation. Try to adjust the light levels and temperature according to her needs, and remember to aerate the area as much as possible, although without causing her to feel cold.

Keeping busy

Where possible, try to keep the person motivated with things that have held lasting interest for her. This might mean encouraging suitable pastimes that she can enjoy, such as listening to a favourite radio programme, or you could go through photo albums together, or read out extracts of old letters. If she is up to it, try to encourage short visits from friends and family – lengthy visits may overwhelm and tire her out. Be ready to cancel any plans if she does not feel up to it on the day.

Personal care

Try to enable the person to present herself physically as she would have done in the past, for example by applying lipstick,

brushing her hair, keeping her nails trimmed, or tidying her clothes. Small details such as these can be very important as they help to maintain the person's dignity as well as her quality of life.

Encouraging eating

As the person you care for withdraws, she will probably lose her appetite and begin to lose weight, which will affect how she looks and the way her clothes fit. You may notice she now seems to be aging and her skin colour may change slightly.

While you can't force her to eat, you can try to encourage her appetite. Try making her portions of food a little smaller, but

CONTROLLING PAIN

Not everyone who is dying experiences pain, but if it is a problem there are effective ways to help control it (see pp.162–163 for more information).

- Doctors and nurses are skilled at giving painkillers that reduce suffering while minimizing side effects.

- You may be able to improve the person's pain by applying warmth or cold to the area of discomfort or by repositioning her.

- Complementary therapies, such as acupuncture, are found to be effective by some people.

- A pain-relieving device, such as a TENS machine, may help provide pain relief.

offer snacks more regularly, and make an effort to focus on foods or dishes you know she favours. Appetite stimulants are also worth trying. For example, the smell of vanilla can stimulate the appetite, as can a small glass of wine or other alcoholic drink before food, although you should first check with the person's doctor whether this is okay. Nutritious high-calorie drinks are good for boosting a person's nutrient intake when her appetite is small.

The important thing to remember is to discuss any concerns with a medical professional, who may be able to offer suggestions and reassure you.

Comfort aids

Some people in the dying phase put on weight due to fluid retention, causing swelling in the feet and legs. In order to keep the person comfortable, you may need to use additional equipment, such as elastic stockings to reduce foot and leg swelling or a footstool to keep her feet elevated and allow excess fluid to drain away. The doctor may suggest gentle exercises to help to relieve the swelling.

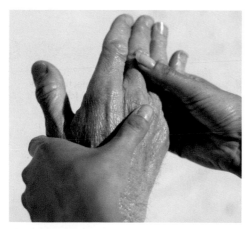

Alleviating dry skin
Gently massaging moisturizer into the skin of the person relieves any uncomfortable dryness, and also helps stimulate her circulation.

> ### LOOK OUT FOR SYMPTOMS OF INFECTION
>
> It is important as a carer to be aware that infections are more common in the dying phase, and if you think the person you are caring for is gradually or suddenly becoming unwell, call the doctor. Key symptoms to look out for include running a high temperature, shivering, or shaking.

The last few days of life

As the person enters the last few days of life, she will need a lot more physical care. The specialist nurse will be able to show you how to adapt your care techniques and what extra things you may have to do and consider during the last few days.

As the final hours approach, you'll notice signs that death is near. The person will become weaker and will sleep for longer periods; she may slip in and out of consciousness; or she may just be awake but not want, or be able, to speak. For many people the last few hours are calm and peaceful, but it can be a frightening experience for the carer as you anticipate the worst. Try to focus on keeping the person as comfortable as possible.

■ **Skin care** The person's skin will need moisturizing frequently to prevent any discomfort and damage from dryness, and you may need to ask someone to help you to wash her properly. She is unlikely to be able to turn over on her own, so you may have to help reposition her every few hours to prevent the development of pressure sores (p.102), which are caused by lying in the same position. See pp.113–115 for practical advice on how to turn a person safely and comfortably.

■ **Mouth care** You may need to give more frequent mouth care, using swabs to moisten and clean the mouth area and applying lip moisturizer, especially if she is not able to swallow fluids well any more. The specialist nurse can show you how to do this and will get any mouth and skin care supplies needed from the person's doctor. Having a refreshed mouth and moisturized lips can bring much comfort.

■ **Keeping warm** In the last few hours before death, the person's hands and feet may feel cold or clammy and may look a different colour with a bluish tinge. You can keep her comfortable with cosy socks and light blankets or a sheet.

■ **Talk and touch** Most people slip into unconsciousness, and you may find you are unable to wake her up and may worry she can't hear you when you talk. However, hearing is thought to be the last sense to go, so try to speak reassuringly and calmly to the person. You may be able to read to her, play some favourite music, or simply sit quietly and hold her hand or gently rub her skin to accompany her through this stage. For the person it is very comforting to know someone is nearby.

■ **Spiritual support** Depending on the person's belief system, in the last few days of her life you may decide to have prayers recited by a religious or spiritual leader who is close to the person, or by family members. Certain religions have well-structured religious rituals that are both comforting to the person and supportive to you, the carer, especially if you know this was a wish of the one who is now dying. She may want to have religious objects, such as a prayer book, close by for comfort.

Final moments

In the last moments of a person's life, her breathing pattern will change: it may slow down and become irregular, or it may become noisy and bubbly as extra secretions collect and she can't cough or swallow so easily. It may well not be at all distressing for the person, but may be hard for you to watch and listen to. Gradually her breaths will have longer and longer pauses between them and her stomach muscles

may seem to be working more than her chest muscles. Finally, her breathing will cease entirely. This can take a long time, but it may happen more quickly for some and it is hard to predict. After she has stopped breathing, her body and her facial expressions will relax and she is likely to look very peaceful.

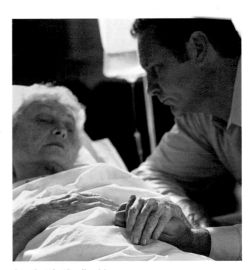

Comfort in the final hours
Staying close to the person in her final few hours is very important. Holding her hand and talking gently will reassure and comfort her.

PRACTICALITIES AFTER DEATH

The days after death can be surprisingly busy as many people must be contacted – not only friends and family but also official organizations. For example, you will need to register the person's death, make the funeral arrangements, and contact all the agencies that need to know she has died. As the carer there may be jobs that you wish to do yourself, but bear in mind that all these tasks can be less onerous if you accept help from other people who wish to be involved. You will feel relieved, and they will feel that they have been able to take away some of your burden.

Who to call first

First of all, the person's doctor needs to be informed that death has occurred – the specialist nurses may do this for you if they are present. The doctor will then come as soon as possible to verify the person has died. You will also need to notify the funeral director, who will come to take the body away to a mortuary until the funeral. Close family may want to spend time alone with the person, and the funeral director will not take the body away until you are all ready.

Certification of death

If the deceased person's doctor has verified the death, he or she may immediately issue a medical certificate stating the cause of death. If, however, the death was verified by another health professional, the doctor will certify the death later, either at the person's home or at the funeral director's.

The doctor certifying the death has a legal responsibility to inform the local coroner, if appropriate – although this is unlikely if the death was expected. A death certificate cannot be issued until the postmortem has been completed.

CHECKLIST OF WHAT NEEDS DOING

The process of arranging the affairs of a person after death can be overwhelming. A simple checklist helps to focus on what is key:

- Inform the person's doctor, who will need to verify and certify the death.
- Call immediate family, who may wish to spend time with the deceased.
- Inform the funeral director, who will collect the body at a time of your choosing.
- Register the death within five days (eight in Scotland). This will provide you with documents you need for a funeral. Ask for several copies of the death certificate.
- In the UK, contact the Department for Work and Pensions to cancel any benefits or allowances the person may have had.
- Arrange the person's funeral.

Arranging the funeral

You may have discussed the funeral with the person before she died, in which case you will know what kind of service she wanted. If not, it can be decided as a family. The funeral director will discuss options with you and then contact the chosen place of burial to arrange a date. If you have chosen a religious funeral, you will also be advised by the leaders of that religion. You may opt for a non-religious service, or may hold a small service for family and then arrange a memorial service for others.

If the person is to be cremated, you will need to take advice from the funeral director as to what can be done with the person's ashes. They cannot just be scattered anywhere, as some locations require formal permission or a licence.

Some families may decide to bury their loved ones abroad, for example in the country of origin, in which case specialist funeral directors and travel agencies will offer advice and support in this process.

BEREAVEMENT

Once the funeral is over, you may find it harder to cope because there are no longer any arrangements keeping you busy. You may feel very lonely for a time as your routine will have changed radically and the days may feel very empty. Allow friends and family to come over or take you out so that you can gradually resume and enjoy other activities while treasuring special memories of the person you cared for.

Reactions to loss

Feeling upset and tearful, angry, numb, or desperate are all normal reactions to loss. You may feel angry that the she has died and left you, or angry that you were unable to prevent her from dying. Missing her can be overwhelming, and from time to time you may experience a strong sense of her presence, or have vivid dreams about her.

Support from others

Talking to others about your feelings can be very cathartic and can help you through the grieving process. Try not to be alone as having people around you can be greatly supportive and allows you to talk when you want to about your loss. It may be helpful to express anxieties about the future as well as to talk about those last precious days and moments with the person you loved.

Remembering

Each time you recollect and remember verbally all the pictures and memories you have in your head, it is helping you to travel through your bereavement. Revisiting the person's room or home or viewing her possessions will help you recall her more vividly, and enable you, gradually, to come to terms with the fact that she has died.

LOOKING AFTER YOURSELF

While your mind and body reel from the profound and significant loss you have incurred, it can be easy to neglect your health and wellbeing. It may be helpful to try to keep busy to fill the hole in your life, but it is also important that you focus attention on yourself and allow yourself time to heal.

- Don't expect too much from yourself. Give yourself permission to be disorganized and make mistakes for a while.

- Look after your health. Lack of sleep and nourishment may mean that you're more prone to infections and illness.

- Try to take some form of exercise, even just gentle walking. It will help release your natural endorphins and energize your body.

- Avoid turning to alcohol – it may result in a dependence if drinking becomes habitual.

- Avoid sleep medication. For the first few days tablets may help you sleep, but in the long term you can become reliant.

- Treat yourself kindly. Try to do one thing extra for yourself each week, such as buying a bunch of flowers or going to the cinema.

- Deal with your feelings. Try writing down your feelings, or sharing them with other members of the family who share your loss.

- Recall happy memories. Remembering the good times with the person who died can be painful but healing. Looking at photographs, making a memory book, and keeping meaningful mementos may help.

- Don't rush to dispose of the peron's clothing – there's no point in giving yourself unnecessary pain at this point. Wait until you feel ready, perhaps keeping a special item that reminds you of the loved one.

- Take things slowly. Don't make any big life changes, such as moving house, starting a new relationship, or changing your job for at least six months. You need time to adjust.

- See p.216 for sources of further help and advice.

11

RESOURCES

■ LEGAL AND FINANCIAL MATTERS ■ USEFUL CONTACTS ■ GLOSSARY

LEGAL AND FINANCIAL MATTERS

Needing to be cared for or taking on the role of carer represents a significant change in circumstances that brings various legal and financial considerations. For older people in particular, changes to their health or income are likely to raise concerns. Carers' concerns may include not only ensuring that personal issues, such as employment rights, are taken care of, but also that they can help look after the affairs of the person they are caring for.

This section deals with the most common issues that may arise and gives guidance on the options that are available and how to get further advice. The information applies to England. Much also applies to Scotland, Wales, and Northern Ireland, although there are some differences in these regions. **While the information here is accurate at the time of publication, legal and financial advice may change over time. If you require legal advice or other expert help, you should seek the services of a competent professional.**

IF YOU ARE THE PERSON NEEDING CARE

Being cared for has several financial implications. You may be unable to work, or be limited in the work you can do; or you may have extra expenses, such as buying specialist equipment. It is vital that you know what benefits and allowances you are entitled to, and that you understand other aspects of financial management, such as how to maximize your savings and deal with tax. If you are concerned you may become unable to manage your financial and other affairs, it is important to be proactive. For example, if you need to make a will or legally nominate someone to manage your affairs for you, take steps to

do this now. By setting things in place you can be confident that your affairs will be managed according to your wishes. Seeking advice from experts can help the process seem more manageable as they will be able to advise you on what issues you may be facing and how best to tackle them.

Benefits and allowances

If you are over a certain age, you will be entitled to basic government allowances, such as state pension (if you have paid or been credited with National Insurance contributions), and there are extra allowances if you are on a low income. These are set out in the table opposite (continued on p.206). There are also allowances for people who require care or who are unable to work because of disability or sickness (pp.206–207).

■ **Means testing** Some benefits and allowances are means tested, which means that you will only receive the benefit if an assessment shows that you could not cope financially without it. Non-means tested benefits are not dependent on a person's financial position.

■ **Terms of benefits** The amount of money offered as a benefit or allowance is subject to change from the government, so specific amounts are not included in this table. The qualifying criteria for benefits may also change. For information on specific amounts to which you may be entitled and the criteria that apply, refer to the government website (p.216).

From October 2013, Universal Credit replaces many means-tested benefits, including Housing Benefit and Working Tax Credit. Those who are already in receipt of these benefits will be gradually reassessed and, if appropriate, moved onto Universal Credit by 2017.

AGE- AND INCOME-RELATED BENEFITS AND ALLOWANCES

BENEFIT/ ALLOWANCE	WHAT IS IT?	PRINCIPAL QUALIFYING CRITERIA
State pension (non-means tested)	■ A regular payment to those who have reached state pension age and have paid or been credited with National Insurance contributions.	■ The amount of pension is based on the number of years of National Insurance contributions you have paid or been credited with.
Pension Credit (means tested)	■ A supplement to the state pension that comes in two separate parts: Guarantee Credit and Savings Credit. Each part increases your weekly income by a certain amount, but the amount you get differs depending on whether you are single or part of a couple.	■ Guarantee Credit – the minimum age is 60–65, depending on your date of birth. If you are disabled, care for someone, or have housing costs, such as mortgage interest, you may be entitled to more. ■ Savings Credit – you must be 65 or over and have made provision for your retirement, such as savings or a second pension.
Winter fuel payment (non-means tested)	■ A payment to ensure older people keep warm during the winter.	■ If you are 60 or over. ■ The annual amount increases for people over the age of 80.
Cold weather payment (means tested)	■ Payments are available if the weather is (or is expected to be) an average of 0°C or lower for seven days in a row.	■ If you receive Pension Credit or certain other means-tested benefits you will automatically receive this payment.
Housing Benefit (means tested)	■ A benefit to assist people who cannot afford their rent.	■ If you are a tenant and receive Guarantee Credit (part of Pension Credit). ■ If you are a tenant on a low income with savings/assets below a fixed amount. ■ If you claim Attendance Allowance, Disability Living Allowance, or Carer's Allowance this may increase the amount of Housing Benefit you can receive.
Council Tax Benefit (means tested) and other reliefs from Council Tax (non-means tested)	■ Benefits and/or reliefs that reduce your Council Tax bill.	■ If you receive the Guarantee Credit (part of Pension Credit) or if you have low income and low savings/assets. ■ Reductions may apply if your property is unoccupied; if your home has been adapted for a disabled person; if an occupant is mentally impaired; or if you are the only occupant. ■ Local authorities can also make discretionary discounts to your Council Tax.

AGE- AND INCOME-RELATED BENEFITS AND ALLOWANCES

BENEFIT/ ALLOWANCE	WHAT IS IT?	PRINCIPAL QUALIFYING CRITERIA
The Social Fund (means tested)	■ Offers loans and grants for extra costs, including crisis loans; community care grants; energy efficiency grants; budgeting loans; and cold weather payments.	■ These are available for people on low incomes and with low savings/ assets, including those in receipt of Guarantee Credit (part of Pension Credit). Different conditions apply for each scheme.
NHS health benefits (non-means tested)	■ Free NHS dental treatment, NHS eye tests, and NHS prescriptions. ■ A voucher towards the cost of glasses or contact lenses. ■ Payment towards travel costs to attend NHS treatment.	■ These are automatically available if you receive Guarantee Credit (part of Pension Credit). ■ If you are over 60, you get free prescriptions and free eye tests.
Travel benefits (non-means tested)	■ A Senior Railcard can be bought, entitling you to one third off most rail fares in Great Britain. ■ An English National Concessionary Travel Scheme (ENCTS) bus pass entitles you to free travel at most times of the day on local buses in England outside London. ■ A Freedom Pass entitles you to free travel on almost all public transport in London at most times of the day.	■ For a Senior Railcard, you must be 60 or over. ■ For an ENCTS bus pass, you must have reached the state pension age of a woman with your date of birth. If you have a Freedom Pass, you do not need to apply separately for an ENCTS bus pass. ■ For a Freedom Pass, your main residence must be in London and you must have reached the state pension age of a woman with your date of birth.
Direct payments (means tested)	■ Payments from the local authority to enable you to buy community care services. They cannot be used to pay for permanent residential care.	■ If you are assessed as needing community care services and have a low income and low savings/assets.

DISABILITY AND SICKNESS BENEFITS AND ALLOWANCES

BENEFIT/ ALLOWANCE	WHAT IS IT?	PRINCIPAL QUALIFYING CRITERIA
Attendance Allowance (non-means tested)	■ A non-taxable benefit for people who are physically or mentally disabled and require care.	■ You may qualify if you have had care needs or mobility problems for six months and are over 65. The qualifying period may be waived if you are terminally ill. ■ Paid at a lower rate for those who need care by day or by night; a higher rate is paid for those who need care both day and night.

DISABILITY AND SICKNESS BENEFITS AND ALLOWANCES

BENEFIT/ ALLOWANCE	WHAT IS IT?	PRINCIPAL QUALIFYING CRITERIA
Disability Living Allowance (non-means tested)	■ A non-taxable benefit for people who are physically or mentally disabled and require care. ■ From April 2013, the Personal Independence Payment (see below) replaces DLA. If you were already receiving DLA before this date, your payment may change.	■ You may qualify if you have had care needs or mobility problems for three months, you are likely to need help for a further six months, and you are under 65 when you apply. The qualifying periods may be waived if you are terminally ill.
Personal Independence Payment (means tested)	■ A new benefit that replaces Disability Living Allowance from April 2013. ■ Includes a daily living component and a mobility component, each available at two different levels.	■ You may qualify if you have had care needs or mobility problems for three months, you are likely to need help for a further nine months, and you are under 65 when you apply. The qualifying periods may be waived if you are terminally ill.
Disabled Facilities Grants; the Independent Living Fund (both means tested)	■ Grants from your local authority to help you adapt your home to your needs.	■ If you are physically disabled and have a low income and low savings/assets.
Working Tax Credit (means tested)	■ Tax credit (payments) from the government.	■ If you work at least 16 hours a week, are disabled, on a low income, and have low savings/assets.
Statutory Sick Pay	■ A fixed weekly rate payable by your employer for the first 28 weeks of illness.	■ If you are an employee earning over a certain amount per week and are off work due to sickness
Employment and Support Allowance (ESA)	■ Financial, government-funded support for those who cannot work because of sickness or disability and are not receiving Statutory Sick Pay. There are two types of allowance: Contributory ESA and Income-related ESA.	■ Contributory ESA may be available if you have paid enough National Insurance contributions. ■ Income-related ESA may be available if both your income and savings/assets are below certain levels. An assessment will check you have a limited ability to work.
Travel benefits (non-means tested)	■ A Disabled Person's Railcard can be bought, entitling you to one third off most rail fares in Great Britain. ■ An English National Concessionary Travel Scheme (ENCTS) bus pass (see opposite). ■ A Freedom Pass (see opposite).	■ For a Disabled Person's Railcard, you must have one or more specified disabilities or receive a disability-related allowance. ■ For an ENCTS bus pass or Freedom Pass, you must have one or more specified disabilities. For a Freedom Pass, your main residence must be in London.

Managing your finances

It's important to try to keep track of your money, in particular being sure of how much you have and how your income compares to your outgoings. Effective management of savings, income, and bill payments is important to ensure that you do not get into financial difficulty.

■ **Savings** If you have modest savings, arrange a meeting with your bank representative to check whether you are getting the best rate of interest on your savings. Check in the financial section of newspapers or online for comparisons of savings accounts with different banks.

■ **Independent financial advice** If you have significant savings or income and have more money coming in than going out, it is generally best to get advice from an Independent Financial Advisor (IFA), who can consider savings and investment products across all the different banks and institutions. An IFA will have to charge you, so ask about their fees at the outset. Check also that your advisor is regulated by the Financial Services Authority (FSA).

■ **Direct debits** These are automatically generated, regular payments made direct from your bank account. Setting these up can help avoid unpaid bills.

■ **Equity release** If you own your own home, this is an asset from which funds can be released by way of a mortgage loan. Some lenders offer loans whereby, as long as you abide by certain conditions, the loan and interest do not need to be repaid until the house is sold or you die. These are referred to as equity release schemes. People sometimes release funds from their home if they want to carry on living there for the foreseeable future but want or need to raise a lump sum of money.

Approach equity release schemes with caution and take advice before entering into one. Although different schemes vary, overall they tend to be an expensive way to borrow as the money is released as a loan and the lenders often charge a relatively high level of interest. You may pay interest not only on the main loan itself, but also on interest for previous years. For this reason, the amount you pay at the end is likely to be much more than the amount originally borrowed.

A financial expert can check for you whether there are other, cheaper ways of raising the money you want or need, for example via government grants, welfare benefits, normal loans, or mortgages.

Dealing with tax

Tax can be a daunting aspect of your finances, and it is worth taking advice if you are unsure of your position. Two key areas to be aware of include:

■ **Tax returns** A tax return is a formal document that provides the goverment's Revenue and Customs department (HMRC) with details of any liability for taxation. You may need to complete a tax return if you have been sent one; if you have annual income taxed at the higher rate; if you have sold an asset (other than your main home) at a gain and you need to report a capital gain; or if you wish to claim tax relief.

■ **Inheritance tax** This is a tax charged on your estate when you die (and on certain lifetime gifts you have made). Everyone has an inheritance tax "nil rate band" – this is a specified amount, and any assets up to that amount are taxed at 0 per cent. In other words, if you own less than that amount in total, your estate will probably not pay any inheritance tax. If, however, you own more than that amount, inheritance tax will be charged on the rest of your assets at 40 per cent, subject to exemptions, reliefs, and other conditions.

Any money that you give to your spouse (or registered civil partner) during your lifetime or via your will is exempt from inheritance tax, provided that the person is domiciled in the UK. Gifts to charity are also exempt. Ask a solicitor to advise you in detail about exemptions.

Paying for care

If you require care in later life there are many considerations to take on board, but one important issue is how your care will be paid for. Staying in a care home can be expensive but there are various funding options available (see table, below). The cost of care in one's own home can vary substantially, depending on the type and the frequency of care needed. If a carer is required for much of the week, this is often more expensive than the cost of a care home, but many people, understandably, still prefer to stay in their own home. The funding options for care in your own home are similar to those for care in a care home. However, if the local authority is funding your care and that care could be less expensive in a care home, they may refuse to pay the extra to keep you at home.

> ### THIRD-PARTY FEE TOP-UPS
>
> There is normally a limit to the amount that your local authority will agree to pay for care home fees, even if you are entitled to be fully funded. Any extra fees required by a care home can be paid by someone else (a third party), such as a family member.

FUNDING OPTIONS FOR CARE HOMES

FUNDING	WHAT DO YOU GET?	PRINCIPAL QUALIFYING CRITERIA
Local authority funding	■ Means-tested funding from a local authority towards care home fees. Depending on the outcome of a financial assessment, the local authority may offer more or less funding, or none. ■ For the initial 12 weeks of living in a care home, the value of your family home will be ignored when the local authority assesses how much money you have.	■ If you are assessed as needing to be looked after in a care home. ■ In most cases, you must not have income or savings/assets over a certain amount or the local authority will not pay towards care home fees. However, national guidelines state when the local authority should assist, set out in the Charging for Residential Accommodation Guide (CRAG), see the government website, p.216).
Deferred payment agreements	■ Payment towards care in a home made by the local authority on your behalf; you will need to repay the amount when your house is sold.	■ The local authority may agree to such an arrangement if you do not have money immediately available but do have an asset such as your house, which you are able to sell.
NHS continuing healthcare	■ An NHS-funded package of care, which may include payment of care home fees, and healthcare and personal care costs.	■ If your primary need for care relates to your need for healthcare, you may qualify for NHS continuing health care.
Section 117 aftercare services	■ Full payment of care costs will be met by the local authority.	■ In extreme circumstances when it has been necessary to detain someone in hospital for treatment under the Mental Health Act 1984.

Giving authority

If you have any concerns regarding your ongoing mental or physical health, a clear way to ensure your affairs are properly looked after is to make a power of attorney. This is the legal authorization that one person (the donor) grants to another (the attorney) to manage his private affairs.

There are various types of power of attorney. A General Power of Attorney (GPA) gives the attorney authority to deal with your financial affairs, but it is automatically revoked if you lose mental capacity (p.212). A Lasting Power of Attorney (LPA) for Property and Financial Affairs grants the authority to deal with some or all of your property and financial affairs, even if you lose mental capacity. An LPA for Health and Welfare grants the authority to deal with your care and health affairs but can only be used if you lose mental capacity. The LPA has, since October 2007, replaced the Enduring Power of Attorney (EPA), except that EPAs made before then will continue to be valid.

People often choose relatives, friends, or carers as their attorneys. You can also appoint a professional advisor, such as a solicitor or accountant, but in that case the attorney will charge for their services.

Making a will

A will is a key document for putting your affairs in order for when you die and will only take effect after your death. As long as you have mental capacity to make a will, your will can be changed and updated as you please. Making a will allows you to:

■ Select who you want to be responsible for managing your affairs after your death.
■ Decide who should inherit your assets.
■ Set up trusts to protect the interests of vulnerable relatives and friends.
■ Record your funeral wishes.
■ Appoint guardians for your children, in case they are still minors when you die.

There are strict rules as to how a will must be made, and if any of them are not followed the will may be invalid. For this reason, when making a will it is worth getting advice from a solicitor. You can only make or alter a will when you still have the mental capacity to do so ("testamentary capacity"), otherwise it will be invalid. Your solicitor can advise you on the legal rules regarding testamentary capacity.

IF YOU ARE A CARER

Providing care for another person can have significant financial implications on your daily living, particularly if your role as a carer forces you to make alterations to the terms of your normal job. Investigate carefully what options are available in order to alleviate financial strain where possible.

Your ability to help with the financial and legal affairs of the person you are caring for will depend on whether they have granted you the authority, known as power of attorney (p.213). Even without this, there are still ways that you can help.

Benefits and entitlements

As a carer you automatically gain certain legal rights that aim to support you in your role as a carer, for example you are entitled to have your needs assessed by your local authority. If you are also in employment you have certain legal rights, such as the right to request flexible working arrangements. In addition to these rights, you may also be entitled to direct financial help.

The table opposite provides details of both your legal and financial entitlements. As the terms of these are subject to government change, payment details have not been included. For further information on specific amounts to which you may be entitled and the qualifying criteria, refer to the government website (p.216).

ALLOWANCES AND RIGHTS FOR CARERS

ENTITLEMENT	WHAT DO YOU GET?	PRINCIPAL QUALIFYING CRITERIA
Carer's Allowance	■ A fixed weekly payment of a specified amount.	■ If you spend at least 35 hours a week caring for a disabled person who receives a qualifying disability benefit. ■ If you are also employed, you can only get Carer's Allowance if your net earnings are under a certain amount.
Carer's Credit	■ This allows you to build up your National Insurance contributions towards a state pension.	■ If you care for someone who is disabled for 20 hours or more per week and are not in receipt of Carer's Allowance.
Local authority needs assessment	■ A carer's assessment will take your needs into account, including travel, daily activities, work commitments, further education, and leisure activities. Based on the outcome, you may be given direct payments (see below). ■ Your local authority will liaise with other local authorities, education authorities, housing authorities, and health organizations to consider requests for services for you or the person being cared for.	■ If you are 16 or over and provide a regular and substantial amount of care for an adult. ■ To request a needs assessment, contact your local social services department.
Direct payments	■ Payments that the local authority can make to you, the carer. ■ Enables you to arrange your own care services rather than relying on social services. ■ Can be used to buy services to support your work as a carer, including courses, extra carer support, or a respite break.	■ If you are assessed as needing help from social services.
Rights at work	■ The right to request flexible working arrangements from your employer. Employers are not obliged to agree but they must provide proper business reasons if they refuse the request. ■ The right to take unpaid leave to care for a dependant in an emergency.	■ If you are a carer and are also in employment. ■ You can request flexible working arrangements if you are the carer of an adult who is a relative and who lives at the same address as you.

HOW CAN A CARER HELP WITH LEGAL AND FINANCIAL MATTERS?

Many carers are in a position where they have no official authority (power of attorney, p.210) to help look after the affairs of the person they are caring for. If this is the case, the extent to which a carer can help will depend on the person's situation.

It may be that the person you are caring for is physically frail but has full mental capacity (see panel, right). In this situation there are a number of practical steps you can take to make life easier, for example helping the person to claim benefits. If the person has lost mental capacity and has not given you power of attorney (p.213), then you are more limited, but there are still ways that you can help.

Accessing government benefits

Most welfare benefits can be applied for via post, phone, or the internet, or by personal application at relevant benefit offices. Even without power of attorney you can help with filling in forms and gathering information. If the person you are caring for has mental capacity, applying for benefits can be quite simple as he can sign his own claim forms.

If you are applying by telephone and have the person with you, he can speak to the advisor first to confirm any details and to authorize the advisor to discuss his affairs with you. However, even if he is not present at the time, if you are able to confirm various personal details the benefits agency will often agree to discuss the benefits you are claiming on his behalf.

■ **Appointees** If you want to look after the benefits of someone who has lost mental capacity and has not appointed an attorney, you can contact the Department of Work and Pensions (DWP) to inform them that you want to become the person's

WHAT IS MENTAL INCAPACITY?

"Mental capacity" is the legal term for the ability of a person to make decisions that affect either himself or other people. People suffering from certain conditions may lose their mental capacity. Such conditions include degenerative diseases, such as dementia, and brain injuries resulting from an accident or a stroke. A person will be deemed to lack mental capacity to make a particular decision if any of the following apply:

- He cannot understand the information needed to make that decision, even if it is presented in a way that is suited to his needs, such as simple language.

- He cannot remember the information long enough to use it.

- He cannot use or evaluate the information in order to make a decision.

- He is unable to communicate his decision in any way.

Legal safeguards are in place for a person who lacks mental capacity, as overseen by the Court of Protection (see panel, right). Any decision made for him must be on the basis of an assessment of his best interests, taking into account any preference he is able to express or has expressed in the past. The Court of Protection can adjudicate on this.

appointee. The DWP will interview you and will also visit the person you are looking after. If the DWP agrees that he needs help and that appointing you is in his best interests, you will be formally appointed.

Paying for care in a care home

If the person you look after needs to move into a care home or to receive professional care support at home, there are some limited ways in which you can help.
- If he has low income and savings/assets, you can help him request a financial assessment from the local authority.
- If he has severe healthcare needs, ask for an NHS continuing healthcare assessment (p.209) to be carried out.
- If he receives benefits, check that he is receiving everything he is entitled to.

Statutory wills for people who have lost mental capacity

If the person has lost the mental capacity to make a will and has either not made a will or his current will needs updating, you can apply to the Court of Protection (see panel, right) to ask the court to approve a new will for the person. This is called a statutory will. Because there are specific requirements for the court application, it is best to seek advice on this from a solicitor.

Carers with power of attorney

There are several different types of power of attorney, and the type you have will determine which aspects of a person's affairs you have the authority to manage.

■ **Lasting Power of Attorney (LPA) for Health and Welfare** This LPA gives you the authority to make decisions about a person's care and medical treatment, but only comes into force once the person has lost mental capacity (see p.196 for more detail).

■ **Lasting Power of Attorney (LPA) for Property and Financial Affairs** This LPA enables you to manage a person's money and/or property (subject to any restrictions the person may have specified), whether he has mental capacity or not.

■ **Enduring Power of Attorney (EPA)** The EPA, which enables the attorney to manage the property and financial affairs of a person even if the person loses mental capacity, has now been replaced by the LPA for Property and Financial Affairs. However, if you have a valid EPA dating from before October 2007, you are still able to act on behalf of the person you are caring for.

If you have power of attorney for the person you are caring for and he has lost mental capacity, you will need to rely on your own judgment when making decisions concerning his affairs.

■ **Legal obligations** Any decisions that you make for the person you are helping must

THE COURT OF PROTECTION

The Court of Protection has jurisdiction to make decisions for those who lack mental capacity. If a person has lost mental capacity, it can authorize a deputy to act in that person's best interests, issue a statutory will (left), and settle disputes. The forms required to make an application to the Court of Protection are available via the government website (p.216).

be in his best interests. You must keep accounts and use reasonable care and skill in managing his finances. You must keep the person's money in a separate bank account from your own. If your actions cause financial loss, you can be personally responsible for compensating that loss. Unless you are acting as a professional attorney (normally a solicitor or an accountant), you cannot accept any payment. However, you may be reimbursed for expenses that you incur in your duties.

■ **Checking the LPA/EPA is valid** An LPA is only valid once it has been registered and stamped by the Office of the Public Guardian. Only you (as attorney) or the person who appointed you can apply for registration. You will need to use the prescribed form for registration, which can be found on the government website (p.216). When applying to register, you will need to send a formal notice to anyone that the LPA states should be notified.

If you have an EPA, check that it was signed before October 2007, otherwise it is not valid. If the person who made the EPA is losing mental capacity, you will need to register the EPA with the Office of the Public Guardian. Relevant forms are on the government website (p.216).

■ **Ending or cancelling an LPA or EPA** The attorney's control over the person's affairs ends when he dies. As long as the person who made the LPA or EPA still has mental capacity he has the right to revoke that power of attorney at any time.

USEFUL CONTACTS

GENERAL SUPPORT GROUPS

Age UK
www.ageuk.org.uk
Tel: 0800 169 6565

In Wales
www.ageuk.org.uk/cymru
Tel: 0800 169 6565

In Scotland
www.ageuk.org.uk/scotland
Tel: 0845 125 9732

In Northern Ireland
www.ageuk.org.uk/northern-ireland
Tel: 0808 808 7575

Carers Direct
A free advice line for carers.
Tel: 0808 802 0202

Carers UK
www.carersuk.org
Tel: 0808 808 7777

In Northern Ireland
Tel: 02890 439 843

Caring with Confidence
www.caringwithconfidenceonline.co.uk

GENERAL HEALTH

National Institute for Health and Clinical Excellence (NICE)
www.nice.org.uk
Tel: 0845 003 7780

NHS Choices
www.nhs.uk

NHS Direct
www.nhsdirect.nhs.uk
Tel: 0845 4647

In Wales
www.nhsdirect.wales.nhs.uk

In Scotland
www.nhsinform.co.uk
Tel: 0800 22 44 88

In Northern Ireland
www.nidirect.gov.uk

Health Scotland
www.healthscotland.com

CARE HOMES

Care Quality Commission
Regulates health and social care services in England and provides lists of care homes.
www.cqc.org.uk

NHS Choices
Provides information about choosing a care home.
www.nhs.uk/CarersDirect/guide/practicalsupport/Pages/Carehomes.aspx

DISABILITY

Disability Rights UK
Information and advice on independent living
www.disabilityrightsuk.org
Tel: 0845 026 4748

Disabled Living Foundation
www.dlf.org.uk
Tel: 0845 130 9177

SPECIFIC CONDITIONS

CANCER

CancerHelp UK
cancerhelp.cancerresearchuk.org

Macmillan Cancer Support
Provides practical, medical, and financial help for people with cancer.
www.macmillan.org.uk
Tel: 0808 808 0000

Marie Curie Cancer Care
Organizes a free nursing service that supports people with cancer and their carers.
www.mariecurie.org.uk
Tel: 0800 716 146

DEMENTIA

Alzheimer's Society
www.alzheimers.org.uk
Tel: 0300 222 1122

Dementia UK
www.dementiauk.org
Tel: 0845 257 9406

Coventry and Warwickshire Dementia Portal
Information and links to resources for people with dementia and their carers.
http://www.warwickshire.gov.uk/livingwellwithdementia

HEART/LUNG CONDITIONS
British Heart Foundation
www.bhf.org.uk
Tel: 020 7554 0000
Medical information and support: 0300 330 3311

British Lung Foundation
www.lunguk.org
Tel: 0300 0030 555

INCONTINENCE
Incontinence.co.uk
Website providing information about
incontinence and incontinence products.
www.incontinence.co.uk

LEARNING DIFFICULTIES/MENTAL HEALTH
Mencap
Provides help for people with learning difficulties.
www.mencap.org.uk
Tel: 0808 808 1111

Mental Health Foundation
Provides help and information for people with
mental health problems or learning difficulties.
www.mentalhealth.org.uk_

MULTIPLE SCLEROSIS
Multiple Sclerosis Society
www.mssociety.org.uk
Tel: 0800 800 8000

Multiple Sclerosis Trust
www.mstrust.org.uk
Tel: 0800 032 3839

OSTEOPOROSIS
National Osteoporosis Society
www.nos.org.uk
Tel: 0845 450 0230

PAIN
Pain Concern
www.painconcern.org.uk
Tel: 0300 123 0789

PARKINSON'S DISEASE
Parkinson's UK
www.parkinsons.org.uk
Tel: 0800 800 0303

STOMA
Colostomy Association
www.colostomyassociation.org.uk
Tel: 0800 328 4257

Stomawise
Website providing information and links for people
who have had a colostomy, ileostomy, or urostomy.
www.stomawise.co.uk

Urostomy Association
www.urostomyassociation.org.uk
Tel: 01889 563191

STROKE
Different Strokes
Provides support and help to younger stroke
survivors.
www.differentstrokes.co.uk
Tel: 0845 130 7172

Stroke Association
www.stroke.org.uk
Tel: 020 7566 0300
Textphone: 020 7251 9096

VISION/HEARING IMPAIRMENT
Action for Blind People
Runs the former RNIB resource centres in
England.
www.actionforblindpeople.org.uk
Tel: 0303 123 9999

Action on Hearing Loss (formerly RNID)
www.actiononhearingloss.org.uk
Tel: 0808 808 0123
Textphone: 0808 808 9000
Hearing check phone line: 0844 800 3838
Tinnitus enquiries: 0808 808 6666

Deafblind UK
www.deafblind.org.uk
Tel: 0800 132320

In Wales (Deafblind Cymru)
www.deafblindcymru@deafblind.org.uk

Royal National Institute of Blind People (RNIB)
www.rnib.org.uk
Tel: 0303 123 9999

In Wales (RNIB Cymru)
www.rnib.org.uk/cymru
Tel: 029 2045 0440

In Scotland (RNIB Scotland)
www.rnib.org.uk/scotland
Tel: 0131 652 3140

In Northern Ireland (RNIB Northern Ireland)
www.rnib.org.uk/contactdetails/nireland

Sense
Provides support for people who are deafblind.
www.sense.org.uk
Tel/textphone: 0845 127 0066

» USEFUL CONTACTS

HOME ADAPTATIONS

In England

Care and Repair England
www.careandrepair-england.org.uk

Foundation
www.foundations.uk.com

In Wales

Care and Repair Cymru
www.careandrepair.org.uk

In Scotland

Care and Repair Scotland
www.careandrepairscotland.co.uk

In Northern Ireland

Fold
www.foldgroup.co.uk

HOME SAFETY

Royal Society for the Prevention of Accidents (RoSPA)
www.rospa.com

SPECIALIST EQUIPMENT AND CLOTHING

Ability Superstore
www.abilitysuperstore.com
Tel: 0844 358 1398

Able to Wear
www.able2wear.co.uk
Tel: 0141 775 3738

Ableworld
www.ableworld.co.uk

Adaptawear
www.adaptawear.com
Tel: 0845 643 9492

British Red Cross
Loans and sells medical equipment, such as wheelchairs.
www.redcross.org.uk
Tel: 0844 871 1111

Designed to Care
www.designedtocare.co.uk
Tel: 0845 224 9687

Living Made Easy
www.livingmadeeasy.org.uk
Helpline: 0845 130 9177

EXERCISE/ACTIVITIES

Extend
Arranges exercise classes for older people.
www.extend.org.uk
Tel: 01582 832760

Fit as a Fiddle
Provides physical activity and healthy-eating sessions for older people.
www.fitasafiddle.org.uk

National Association for Providers of Activities for Older People (NAPA)
www.napa-activities.co.uk
Tel: 0300 123 0789

LEGAL AND FINANCIAL MATTERS

Benefits enquiries
www.dwp.gov.uk
Tel: 0800 882200

Citizens Advice Bureau (CAB)
www.adviceguide.org.uk
Tel: 08444 111 444 (England)
Tel: 08444 77 20 20 (Wales)

Court of Protection
www.direct.gov.uk
0300 456 4600
Textphone: 020 7664 7755

Gov.UK
The official government website.
www.gov.uk

NHS Low Income Scheme
www.nhs.uk/healthcosts
Tel: 0845 850 1166 (England, Wales, Scotland)
Tel: 0800 587 8982 (Northern Ireland)

DEATH AND BEREAVEMENT

Cruse
Provides counselling, advice, and information for people who have been bereaved.
www.crusebereavementcare.org.uk
Tel: 0844 477 9400

Samaritans
Offers confidential emotional support to anyone going through a crisis.
www.samaritans.org.uk
Tel: 0845 790 9090

GLOSSARY

Advance decision
Also known as a living will. A document specifying the circumstances under which a person would not want to receive life-sustaining treatment. The person must be mentally competent when the advance decision is made for it to be legally valid.

Advance statement
A statement of a person's preferences regarding his or her health and social care. The statement is not legally binding but may be useful when planning a person's care.

Allergy
Any of various conditions caused by an overreaction of the immune system to a particular substance (called an allergen).

Alzheimer's disease
A progressive deterioration in mental functioning due to degeneration of brain tissue. It is the most common cause of dementia.

Analgesics
Drugs used to relieve pain.

Anaphylactic shock
An extreme, life-threatening allergic reaction.

Angina
A constrictive or strangling pain. The term is most commonly used to mean angina pectoris – chest pain due to impaired blood supply to the heart.

Anticoagulants
Drugs used to inhibit blood clotting.

Asthma
A respiratory disorder in which there is intermittent narrowing of the airways, causing wheezing, breathlessness, and a cough.

Attorney
A person who has the legal authority to make decisions on behalf of someone else.

Blood sugar
Also known as blood glucose, the level of the sugar glucose in the blood. Abnormally high levels are an indication of diabetes mellitus.

BMI (body mass index)
A value that indicates whether a person is a healthy weight, underweight, or overweight. It is calculated by dividing the person's weight in kilograms by the square of his or her height in metres.

Body temperature
Normal body temperature is generally considered to be around 37°C (98.6°F), although this varies between individuals and is also affected by factors such as exercise and time of day. A fever is defined as a body temperature over 38°C (100.4°F), and hypothermia as a temperature under 35.5°C (96°F).

Breakthrough pain
A flare-up of pain that breaks through the effects of analgesic medication or other forms of pain control.

Carotid pulse
The rhythmic beats of blood being pumped by the heart that can be felt through the skin over the carotid artery in the neck.

Catheter
A flexible tube inserted into the body, most commonly to drain fluids (such as urine) or introduce fluids (such as drugs).

Colostomy
A surgical operation in which part of the colon (large bowel) is cut, brought through the surface of the skin on the abdomen, and formed into an artificial opening called a stoma.

Concussion
A brain trauma resulting from an injury to the head that causes temporary unconsciousness.

Corticosteroids
Often known just as steroids, a group of drugs most commonly used to reduce inflammation. They may also be used to control allergies, to suppress the immune system (for example, after transplant surgery), and to treat certain cancers and hormone deficiencies.

Court of Protection (CoP)
In England and Wales, a court that has jurisdiction to make decisions for those who lack mental capacity. It can make decisions on behalf of such people and/or can appoint a deputy to take care of a person's affairs.

Degenerative illness
Any disorder in which there is deterioration and loss of function of a body tissue or organ.

Dehydration
Loss of water from the body or the condition in which the body's water level is abnormally low.

Dementia
A general term for various conditions in which there is progressive deterioration of brain functions, particularly behavioural, cognitive, and intellectual functions.

Deputy
A person appointed by the Court of Protection to look after the affairs of someone who no longer has the mental capacity to do so him- or herself.

Diabetes
Any metabolic disorder in which there is excessive urination and constant thirst. The term is usually used to refer to diabetes mellitus, in which deficient production of the hormone insulin or resistance of body cells to its effects causes high blood sugar levels, which leads to excessive urination as the body eliminates the excess sugar in the urine.

Diastolic blood pressure
The lowest level of blood pressure in the arteries, when the heart is relaxed between heartbeats.

Distal
An anatomical term describing a part of the body that is further away from another part with respect to a central point of reference, such as the trunk; for example, the fingers are distal to the elbow.

Electrolytes
When substances such as sodium chloride (common salt) dissolve in a liquid such as water, they split into their constituent parts (called ions) – sodium ions and chloride ions in the case of sodium chloride. These ions are known as electrolytes. In the body, many important substances, such as sodium, potassium, calcium, and chloride, are in the form of electrolytes.

Emollient
A substance that soothes and softens the skin.

Emphysema
A lung disease in which the walls of the tiny air sacs in the lungs are progressively damaged, reducing the surface area of the lungs and causing increased breathlessness.

Epilepsy
A brain disorder characterized by the tendency to have recurrent seizures.

Hypoallergenic
A term applied to substances that are unlikely to produce an allergic reaction.

Hypoglycaemia
The medical term for low blood sugar level.

Hypothermia
Abnormally low body temperature. It is generally defined as a temperature under 35.5°C (96°F).

Ileostomy
A surgical operation in which the ileum (part of the small intestine) is cut, brought through the surface of the skin on the abdomen, and formed into an artificial opening called a stoma.

Inhaler
A device for administering medication in vapour or powder form.

Insulin
A hormone that regulates levels of the sugar glucose in the blood. Insufficient or no insulin production – or resistance of body cells to its effects – results in diabetes mellitus. Injections of insulin may be used to treat diabetes due to lack of natural insulin.

Intolerance
The inability of a person to take a particular drug without experiencing unacceptable side effects.

Intramuscular
A medical term meaning within a muscle, as in an intramuscular injection, in which a drug is injected into a muscle.

Intravenous
A medical term meaning within a vein, as in an intravenous injection, in which a drug is injected into a vein.

Lasting Power of Attorney (LPA)
There are two forms of LPA: one for health and welfare, which gives an attorney the authority to make decisions about a person's care and medical treatment if that person has lost mental capacity, and one for property and financial affairs, which gives an attorney the authority to manage a person's money and/or property (subject to any restrictions the person may have specified), whether that person has mental capacity or not.

Laxatives
Drugs used to stimulate defecation.

Malnutrition
The condition resulting from insufficient or excessive amounts of certain nutrients and /or calories, or an improper balance of nutrients. Malnutrition may be caused by a poor diet or medical conditions that affect the absorption and/or metabolism of nutrients in the body.

Medication
Any substance used to treat disease.

Meningitis
Inflammation of the meninges (the membranes covering the brain and spinal cord), usually due to infection by bacteria or viruses.

Mental incapacity
In English law, a person is deemed to be mentally incapable of making a decision that affect him- or herself or others if he or she cannot understand the information needed to make that decision; cannot remember the information long enough to use it; cannot use or evaluate the information; or cannot communicate his or her decision.

Metabolism
The collective term for all the chemical processes that take place in the body, The term is also used to refer to the chemical changes that a particular substance or group of related substances (such as carbohydrates) undergo.

Nasogastric tube
A flexible plastic tube that is passed through the nose, down the oesophagus, and into the stomach. It may be used to remove liquids from, or introduce fluids (such as liquid nutrients) into, the stomach.

Nebulizer
A device that converts liquid medication into a mist that can be inhaled through a facemask.

Needlestick injury
Accidental puncture of the skin with a hypodermic needle.

Nutritional supplement
A specially formulated product used to provide additional nutrients and/or calories when a person's diet provides too little of them.

Office of the Public Guardian (OPG)
In England and Wales, an agency whose functions include administing the registration of Lasting Powers of Attorney and Enduring Powers of Attorney and supervising deputies appointed by the Court of Protection.

Opioids
Also sometimes called narcotic drugs, a group of analgesic drugs used to relieve moderate to severe pain. Commonly used opioids include codeine, morphine, and pethidine.

Palliative care
Medical care aimed at relieving symptoms rather than curing the causative disease.

Parenteral nutrition
Feeding through a tube inserted into a vein; also known as intravenous nutrition.

PEG tube
A tube inserted through the skin and into the stomach to enable food, liquids, or medication to be introduced directly into the stomach.

Pessary
Any of a variety of devices placed in the vagina. The term is commonly used to refer to a plug or capsule inserted into the vagina in order to administer medication.

Power of attorney
The legal authorization that one person (called the donor) gives to another (the attorney) to manage his or her private affairs. There are various types of power of attorney, notably an Enduring Power of Attorney and two forms of Lasting Power of Attorney (one for property and financial affairs, the other for health and welfare).

Pressure sores
Also known as decubitus ulcers or bedsores, ulcers that develop on an area of skin due to prolonged pressure on that area.

Proximal
An anatomical term describing a part of the body that is nearer another part with respect to a central point of reference, such as the trunk; for example, the elbow is proximal to the fingers.

Radial pulse
The rhythmic beats of blood being pumped by the heart that can be felt through the skin over the radial artery in the wrist.

Respite care
Help that enables a carer to take a break from looking after the person in his or her care.

Seizure
A sudden episode of abnormal activity in the brain. Recurrent seizures occur in epilepsy.

Shock
A dangerous reduction in blood flow throughout body tissues. The term may also refer to the mental distress that may follow a traumatic experience.

Sleep apnoea
A disorder in which there are episodes of temporary breathing stoppage during sleep.

Spacer
A plastic chamber that fits onto the mouthpiece of an inhaler to make it easier to inhale the medication.

Spasticity
Abnormal rigidity in a group of muscles, causing stiffness and restricted movement.

Sterile
Completely free of germs. The term is also sometimes used to mean infertile.

Stoma
An opening in the skin. A stoma is created surgically during a colostomy or ileostomy to allow intestinal contents to pass out of the body, or during a urostomy to allow urine to pass out.

Stroke
A serious condition that occurs when the blood supply to part of the brain is cut off.

Subcutaneous
A medical term meaning under the skin, as in a subcutaneous injection, in which a drug is injected under the skin.

Suppository
A plug or capsule that is inserted into the rectum to administer medication.

Systolic blood pressure
The highest level of blood pressure, when the heart is contracting during a heartbeat to pump blood through the arteries.

Telecare
The use of technological devices to remotely monitor a person and/or his or her home and to provide an alert if there is a problem, such as the person falling or a fire.

Thyroid disorders
The thyroid gland helps to regulate the rate of all the body's internal processes. If the thyroid is overactive, it may cause symptoms such as rapid heartbeat, sweating, trembling, anxiety, and weight loss. Symptoms of underactivity of the thyroid may include tiredness, poor concentration and memory problems, and weight gain.

Transient ischaemic attack (TIA)
Commonly known as a mini-stroke, a TIA is a temporary interruption in the blood supply to the brain.

Urostomy
A surgical operation in which urine is diverted out of the body through an artificial opening (stoma) created in the abdominal wall.

INDEX

INDEX AND ACKNOWLEDGMENTS

221

ACKNOWLEDGMENTS

The publishers would like to thank:

Jane Parker for the index; Nikky Tywman for proofreading; Allan Clarke, Carol Rhind and all the staff at Bucklesham Grange Care Home, Ipswich for the use of facilities for photoshoots; Rose Health Care Centre, Ipswich for the loan of equipment; Julia Phipps at Specialist Mobility for images; Ann Peters RGN, HV for additional consultancy

For modelling: Michelle Baxter, Kaiya Shang, Frances Hewson, Colin Brewster, Spencer Holbrook, Jonathan Metcalf, Janet Mohun, Jenny Pattison, Shirley Cook, Moira Ellice, Sharon Harvey, Julie Stewart, Richard Barrett, Athene Barrett, Demii Hart, Michael Spencer, Patrick Sweeney, Sheila Spencer, Harvey Keys, Valerie Baxter, Lynda Sweeney, Nigel Wright

The publisher would like to thank the following for their kind permission to reproduce their photographs:

(Key: a-above; b-below/bottom; c-centre; f-far; l-left; r-right; t-top)
2 Getty Images: Rob Lewine 11 Getty Images: the Agency Collection / Silvia Jansen. 13 Corbis: David Harrigan / ableimages. 14 Corbis: Dann Tardif / LWA. 15 Patterson Medical: (cb). 16 Dorling Kindersley: Alexander Raths / Shutterstock. 22 Getty Images: Cultura / Hybrid Images. 25 Corbis: JLPH / Cultura. 28 Getty Images: Cultura / Nils Hendrik Mueller. 30 Patterson Medical: (cr, br). 31 Patterson Medical: (br). 32 Patterson Medical. 33 Platinum Stairlifts / Platinum Rails. 35 Patterson Medical: (tl). 37 Patterson Medical: (tl, ftr, fcra/t, fcra/c, fcra/b, fcr, cr, fcrb, fbr). 39 Patterson Medical. 41 Patterson Medical: (tr). 46 Dorling Kindersley: Sarah Ashun (fbr). 55 Patterson Medical: (fcr, c, fcrb, bc). 57 Alamy Images: Viktor Fischer. 61 Corbis: Ariel Skelley. 66 Corbis: Maskot. 69 Patterson Medical: (cla, tr, cl, fcl, clb). 70 Corbis: JGI / Tom Grill / Blend Images. 71 Getty Images: Photonica / Silvia Otte (bl). Patterson Medical: (tr). 72 Getty Images: Stockbyte / altrendo images. 78 Corbis: Terry Vine / Blend Images. 79 PunchStock: Purestock. 87 Patterson Medical: (cla, cl). 88 Patterson Medical: (cra, cl, clb, crb). 106 Corbis: Jose Luis Pelaez Inc. / Blend Images. 110 Patterson Medical: (tr, cr). 111 Patterson Medical. 119 Patterson Medical. 121 Patterson Medical: (cr, cl, crb, br). 122 Patterson Medical. 124 Corbis: Blue Jean Images. 129 Patterson Medical. 134 Patterson Medical. 135 Patterson Medical: (tl, br). 136 Patterson Medical: (tl, crb, br). 138 Patterson Medical: (fbl, bl, br, fbr). 139 Patterson Medical. 148 Corbis: Adam Gault / Science Photo Library. 151 Getty Images: Taxi / Garry Wade. 153 Corbis: Laura Doss. 155 Getty Images: Altrendo Images. 157 Corbis: Sean Justice. 159 Corbis: Kristopher Grunert. 163 Science Photo Library: Simon Fraser, Hexham General. 164 Corbis: Herry Choi / TongRo Images. 166 Science Photo Library. 167 Corbis: Ian Hooton / Science Photo Library. 168 Alamy Images: Dennis Hallinan. 192 Getty Images: Adam Gault / SPL. 195 Corbis: Ian Lishman / Juice Images. 198 Corbis: Bernd Vogel. 199 Corbis: FK Photo.

All other images © Dorling Kindersley
For further information see: www.dkimages.com